BEGINNER'S

GUIDE TO

LOW-HISTAMINE DIET

"A Step-by-Step Plan for Managing Histamine Intolerance, Reducing Inflammation, and Boosting Wellness Naturally"

Anita F. MS RDN McCluskey

Disclaimer

The recipes and information provided in the "Beginner's Guide to Low-Histamine Diet" are meant for educational and informational purposes only. They are not intended to replace professional medical advice, diagnosis, or treatment. If you have any concerns about your health or medical conditions, always seek the guidance of your physician or other qualified healthcare provider. The author and publisher of this book are not responsible for any negative effects or outcomes that may result from using the information or recipes provided. Always prioritize the advice of your healthcare professional when making dietary or health-related decisions.

CONTENT

Introduction

Welcome to the "Beginner's Guide to the Low-Histamine Diet," where healing begins with nourishing food. I'm Anita F. McCluskey, and I've created this cookbook to provide simple, easy-to-follow recipes specifically designed for those managing histamine intolerance, a condition in which the body struggles to break down histamine. Having witnessed firsthand the positive impact of dietary changes in managing this condition, I've compiled a variety of recipes aimed at reducing histamine levels, promoting gut health, and improving overall wellness.

For those with histamine intolerance, managing histamine levels is key to achieving optimal health. The right foods can regulate histamine production and reduce the strain on your body. This cookbook offers flavorful, nutritious meals that not only support living with histamine intolerance but also empower you to thrive.

Drawing from my personal experience and research, I've carefully crafted recipes using ingredients that assist the body in managing histamine. I encourage you to explore this cookbook and embark on your journey toward better health, knowing that every meal you prepare brings you closer to healing.

Real-Life Stories of Low-Histamine Diet Success

Emily Roberts, a 35-year-old graphic designer from Florida, struggled for years with fatigue, skin issues, and digestive discomfort before discovering she had histamine intolerance. Her symptoms included headaches, rashes, and persistent discomfort. It wasn't until she understood how diet could impact her condition that her life started to improve.

"Once I realized how much my diet could affect my histamine intolerance, I felt empowered to take control of my health," Emily shares. "By incorporating low-histamine foods and supporting my body's natural ability to process histamine, I've seen a significant transformation. I now have more energy, fewer flare-ups, and my skin has greatly improved."

Emily enjoys meals like Fresh Herb Chicken, which is gentle on the body and free from high-histamine ingredients, and Sweet Potato & Zucchini Stir-Fry, known for supporting gut health. Her experience illustrates how a thoughtful diet can be essential for managing histamine intolerance.

Her story proves how even small dietary adjustments can make a big difference. "If you're dealing with histamine intolerance, a well-planned meal plan is essential for taking control of your health," Emily says. "It's been life-changing for me."

Michael Johnson, a 48-year-old construction worker from New Jersey, was diagnosed with histamine intolerance after years of unexplained fatigue, digestive issues, and mood swings. The physical toll was significant, but the emotional and mental strain was just as challenging.

"I didn't realize how powerful food could be in managing histamine intolerance until I started using recipes designed to reduce histamine," Michael explains. "I've always enjoyed cooking, but I never understood how to adjust my meals for my health. Once I embraced this diet, I started feeling like myself again—more energetic, with less discomfort and sharper mental clarity."

Michael's favorite meals include Cucumber and Avocado Salad (packed with fresh, low-histamine ingredients) and Grilled Chicken with Olive Oil (renowned for its anti-inflammatory properties). His approach to food has been instrumental in regaining control over his health.

"This shows that making informed food choices can lead to healing," he says. "This cookbook demonstrates how simple it can be to make these changes. I hope it inspires others facing histamine intolerance to take charge of their health."

How This Cookbook Can Support Your Journey to Better Health

The experiences of Emily and Michael highlight the profound impact that thoughtful dietary choices can have in managing histamine intolerance. By incorporating the right foods, they have alleviated the effects of the condition and improved their overall well-being. Their stories show that with the right nutrition—like the recipes in this cookbook—you can transform your health.

As you embark on this journey with this cookbook, rest assured that every recipe has been carefully designed to support your histamine levels, enhance your health, and help you live a vibrant, fulfilling life. Each meal you prepare is a step toward better health and taking control of your wellness.

Let these recipes guide you toward thriving with histamine intolerance!

Understanding low-histamine

Low histamine refers to a condition where the body has insufficient histamine levels, a substance that plays key roles in immune function, stomach acid regulation, and neurotransmission. When histamine levels are too low, it can cause various symptoms and effects. This condition is less common than high histamine levels, which are seen in disorders like histamine intolerance and allergic reactions.

Types of Low Histamine Conditions:

1. Histamine Deficiency:
This rare condition occurs when the body doesn't produce enough histamine. It may be due to factors like genetic issues

or enzyme deficiencies (e.g., diamine oxidase deficiency).

2. DAO Deficiency (Diamine Oxidase Deficiency):

DAO is the enzyme responsible for breaking down histamine in the digestive system. A deficiency in this enzyme can lead to a disruption in histamine metabolism, resulting in low histamine levels.

Symptoms of Low Histamine:

1. Fatigue:

Since histamine influences wakefulness and energy, low levels can cause persistent tiredness or difficulty staying awake.

2. Dizziness and Low Blood Pressure:

Histamine helps control blood pressure, and insufficient levels can lead to dizziness, lightheadedness, or fainting.

3. Digestive Issues:
 As histamine aids in producing stomach acid, a deficiency can cause problems like bloating, indigestion, or constipation.

4. Allergic-like Reactions:
Surprisingly, low histamine levels can sometimes mimic allergy symptoms like itching or rashes, though without the typical inflammatory response seen with high histamine levels.

5. Headaches and Migraines:
While high histamine levels are often linked to headaches, low levels can also cause headaches due to disrupted neurotransmitter regulation.

6. Cognitive Issues:
Histamine functions as a neurotransmitter in the brain, so low levels can lead to brain fog, trouble concentrating, or memory problems.

7. Mood Disturbances:

Histamine is involved in mood regulation, and a deficiency can contribute to feelings of depression or irritability.

Causes of Low Histamine

1. Genetic Factors:

Some people may inherit genetic mutations that affect their ability to produce or process histamine, leading to lower levels.

2. DAO Enzyme Deficiency:

A shortage of diamine oxidase (DAO), the enzyme that breaks down histamine, can cause imbalances in histamine levels in different parts of the body.

3. Chronic Stress

Long-term stress can alter the body's biochemistry, potentially leading to reduced histamine production.

4. Medications:

Certain drugs, like antihistamines or corticosteroids, can reduce histamine levels by interfering with its production or function.

5. Nutritional Deficiencies:

A diet lacking essential nutrients such as vitamin B6, copper, and magnesium, which support histamine production, may lead to low histamine levels.

6. Hormonal Imbalances:

Hormonal fluctuations, particularly in estrogen and progesterone levels, can affect histamine synthesis, with lower estrogen potentially reducing histamine production.

Effects of Low Histamine

1. Weakened Immune System

Since histamine is crucial for immune responses, a deficiency can impair the body's ability to fight infections or allergens.

2. Digestive Problems:

Low histamine may reduce stomach acid production, leading to digestive issues like indigestion, bloating, and poor nutrient absorption.

3. Mental Health Effects:

Histamine influences neurotransmitter activity, so low levels can negatively impact mood, cognition, and sleep, potentially leading to anxiety, depression, or sleep disorders.

4. Reduced Alertness and Performance:

As histamine helps maintain alertness and focus, low levels may result in mental fog, poor concentration, and slower cognitive performance.

Managing Low Histamine:

Dietary Changes: Consuming a balanced diet that supports histamine production, including foods rich in vitamin C, B6, and copper, can help.

Supplements: In some cases, taking supplements like vitamin B6 or DAO enzyme may alleviate symptoms.

Medications: Depending on the cause, medications such as antihistamines (for histamine metabolism issues) or hormone replacement therapy (for hormonal imbalances) may be prescribed.

Given the rarity of low histamine conditions, it's important to consult a healthcare provider for proper diagnosis and treatment of symptoms.

The Role of Diet in Managing Histamine Intolerance

Diet plays a significant role in controlling histamine intolerance. Certain foods can exacerbate symptoms by increasing histamine levels, while others may help reduce overall histamine levels in the body. The main goal is to prevent a histamine buildup and alleviate associated symptoms.

1. Reducing Histamine Intake:

A primary focus of a low-histamine diet is to limit foods that contain high levels of histamine, including fermented, aged, or improperly stored foods. Examples of such foods include aged cheeses, cured meats, and alcoholic beverages, all of which should be limited or avoided.

2. Supporting Histamine Breakdown:

Although diet alone cannot fully regulate histamine levels, some foods can help by supporting the body's ability to break down histamine. Nutrient-rich foods that contain antioxidants, vitamin C, vitamin B6, and anti-inflammatory properties can assist in alleviating symptoms.

3. Maintaining Gut Health:

Since the gut plays a vital role in histamine metabolism, a healthy digestive system is key to managing histamine intolerance. A diet rich in fiber and gut-friendly foods can enhance digestion and overall health, improving histamine processing.

Key Nutritional Guidelines for a Low-Histamine Diet

To effectively manage histamine intolerance, it's important to follow specific nutritional guidelines:

1. Limit High-Histamine Foods:

- Avoid or limit foods that are known to be high in histamine, such as:
- Aged cheeses (e.g., cheddar, gouda)
- Processed and cured meats (e.g., salami, pepperoni)
- Alcoholic drinks, especially wine and beer
- Vinegar and pickled foods

- Fermented foods (e.g., sauerkraut, kimchi, soy sauce)

2. Incorporate Histamine Blockers:
- Some foods can help block histamine release and promote its breakdown:
- Foods rich in vitamin C (e.g., bell peppers, broccoli, strawberries) may reduce histamine levels.
- Foods high in vitamin B6 (e.g., turkey, potatoes, spinach) can support enzymes responsible for metabolizing histamine.

3. Focus on Anti-Inflammatory and Gut-Health Foods:
Including foods with anti-inflammatory properties, such as turmeric, ginger, and omega-3-rich foods (e.g., flaxseeds, chia seeds), can help soothe symptoms and support the immune system.

4. Increase Fiber Intake:
High-fiber foods like whole grains, vegetables, and low-histamine fruits aid

digestion and may assist in eliminating histamine from the body. Fiber also promotes the growth of beneficial gut bacteria that support histamine breakdown.

5. Avoid Processed and Preserved Foods:

Processed and preserved foods, such as canned or packaged goods, often contain additives that may trigger histamine reactions. It is best to stick with fresh, whole foods.

6. Limit Alcohol and Caffeine:

Both alcohol and caffeine can stimulate histamine release, so reducing or avoiding these beverages can help mitigate symptoms.

Tips for Following a Low-Histamine Diet

Successfully adhering to a low-histamine diet requires planning and consistency. Here are some practical tips:

1. Meal Planning:

Prepare meals in advance to ensure they are low in histamine and balanced. Focus on fresh, whole foods while minimizing high-histamine options.

2. Careful Label Reading:

Always check food labels for ingredients that may trigger histamine reactions, such as vinegar, fermented products, or preservatives. Opt for simple, natural ingredients whenever possible.

3. Separate High-Histamine Foods from Histamine Blockers:

Avoid pairing histamine-rich foods with foods that may reduce or block histamine effects. For example, avoid consuming alcohol with meals, as it can enhance histamine release.

4. Consider Histamine-Reducing Supplements (With Caution):

If recommended by a healthcare provider, you may consider supplements like vitamin C or DAO (diamine oxidase) to support histamine breakdown. Always consult a medical professional before starting any new supplements.

5. Stay Hydrated:
Drinking plenty of water throughout the day helps support overall health and aids in the elimination of histamine.

6. Monitor Symptoms Regularly:
Keep track of your symptoms and dietary choices to determine which foods trigger your histamine intolerance. Consider maintaining a food journal to track patterns and adjust your diet as needed.

How to Use This Cookbook

This cookbook is designed to help people with histamine intolerance manage their condition by providing recipes that follow the dietary guidelines outlined above.

Here's how to use it effectively:

1. Understand the Ingredients:
Each recipe has been carefully developed to minimize histamine intake, focusing on fresh, low-histamine ingredients. Look for recipes that incorporate vegetables, fresh proteins (like chicken or turkey), and gluten-free grains.

2. Customize Recipes to Your Needs:
Many recipes can be adjusted to suit your preferences or specific tolerances. For example, you can substitute vegetables or proteins based on availability or taste.

3. Plan Weekly Menus:
Use the cookbook's meal plans to structure your weekly meals. This will help you stay organized and stick to your low-histamine diet without feeling overwhelmed.

4. Mind Portion Sizes:

Be mindful of portion sizes, especially when consuming higher-calorie foods. Maintaining a healthy weight is important for overall health and well-being.

5. Try New Recipes:

The cookbook offers a variety of dishes, from simple snacks to elaborate meals. Experimenting with new recipes will keep your diet enjoyable and fulfilling while staying within the low-histamine guidelines.

6. Consult Medical Advice:

Before making significant dietary changes, consult with your healthcare provider. This cookbook is designed to support your treatment plan and should complement medical care.

By following these dietary guidelines and utilizing the cookbook, individuals with histamine intolerance can manage their condition, alleviate symptoms, and improve overall well-being. While diet plays a key role in managing histamine intolerance, it should be part of a comprehensive approach that includes medical treatment and ongoing consultation with a healthcare provider.

Chapter 1

Breakfasts for a Low-Histamine Diet

This chapter provides you with a variety of nourishing breakfast ideas tailored for individuals following a low-histamine diet. The focus is on selecting ingredients that are gentle on the body and help reduce histamine buildup. By understanding how to combine low-histamine foods with key nutrients, you'll learn how to create flavorful, easy-to-make breakfasts that support your health while minimizing histamine exposure. With simple recipes and tips, you'll be able to enjoy meals that are both delicious and compatible with a low-histamine lifestyle.

1. Scrambled Eggs with Spinach and Feta

Preparation Time:
- 10 minutes
- Serves: 3

Ingredients:
- 6 large eggs
- 1 cup fresh spinach, chopped
- 1/4 cup feta cheese, crumbled (optional, based on histamine tolerance)
- 1 tsp olive oil or butter
- Salt and pepper to taste

Instructions:
1. Heat olive oil or butter in a non-stick skillet over medium heat.
2. Add spinach and sauté until wilted, about 2 minutes.
3. Crack the eggs into a bowl, whisk, and season with salt and pepper.

4. Pour the eggs into the skillet with spinach, stirring occasionally until scrambled to your liking.

5. If tolerated, top with feta cheese before serving.

<u>Nutritional Info (per serving):</u>

- Calories: 280
- Protein: 20g
- Fat: 22g
- Carbs: 4g
- Fiber: 1g
- Iron: 1.5mg

Tips:

- Spinach is a great low-histamine option, and pairing it with fresh, seasonal ingredients can help minimize histamine exposure.
- If dairy is a concern, skip the feta or use a low-histamine alternative like ricotta cheese.

2. Oatmeal with Berries and Chia Seeds

Preparation Time:

- 5 minutes
- Serves: 3

Ingredients:

- 1 cup rolled oats
- 2 cups water or unsweetened almond milk
- 1/2 cup mixed berries (choose fresh, low-histamine varieties like blueberries or strawberries)
- 1 tbsp chia seeds
- 1 tbsp honey or maple syrup (optional)

Instructions:

1. Bring water or almond milk to a boil in a saucepan.

2. Add oats and reduce heat, cooking for 3-5 minutes until soft.

3. Remove from heat and stir in chia seeds.

4. Top with fresh berries and drizzle with honey or syrup if desired.

Nutritional Info (per serving):

- Calories: 200
- Protein: 5g
- Fat: 8g
- Carbs: 30g
- Fiber: 6g
- Iron: 2mg

Tips:

- Blueberries and strawberries are commonly well-tolerated on a low-histamine diet. Choose fresh over canned varieties.
- Chia seeds are rich in omega-3s and help support anti-inflammatory benefits.

3. Greek Yogurt Parfait with Flaxseeds

Preparation Time:
- 5 minutes
- Serves: 3

Ingredients:
- 1 1/2 cups plain Greek yogurt (low-histamine varieties)
- 1/4 cup flax seeds
- 1/2 cup mixed berries (blueberries, strawberries)
- 1 tbsp honey or agave syrup (optional)

Instructions:
1. Layer Greek yogurt in three bowls.
2. Top with flaxseeds.
3. Add berries and drizzle with honey or syrup if desired.
4. Serve immediately.

<u>**Nutritional Info (per serving):**</u>

- Calories: 150
- Protein: 12g
- Fat: 7g
- Carbs: 15g
- Fiber: 5g
- Iron: 0.9mg

Tips:

- Choose plain, unsweetened Greek yogurt to avoid added preservatives or flavorings that can trigger histamine release.
- Flaxseeds provide fiber and healthy fats that help digestion and reduce inflammation.

4. Quinoa Porridge with Almond Butter

Preparation Time:
- 10 minutes
- Serves: 3

Ingredients:
- 1 cup quinoa
- 2 cups water or almond milk
- 2 tbsp almond butter
- 1 tsp cinnamon
- 1 tbsp honey (optional)
- 1/4 cup chopped nuts (optional)

Instructions:
1. Rinse quinoa under cold water and drain.

2. In a saucepan, combine quinoa and water or almond milk and bring to a boil.

3. Reduce heat and simmer for 10-12 minutes until quinoa is cooked and liquid absorbed.

4. Stir in almond butter, cinnamon, and honey (if desired).

5. Top with nuts or extra cinnamon if preferred.

Nutritional Info (per serving):

- Calories: 250
- Protein: 8g
- Fat: 14g
- Carbs: 30g
- Fiber: 5g
- Iron: 2.5mg

Tips:

- Quinoa is a naturally low-histamine food, making it a perfect choice for your diet.
- Choose almond butter carefully, as some nut butters may contain preservatives that can increase histamine levels.

5. Avocado Toast with a Side of Berries

Preparation Time:
- 10 minutes
- Serves: 3

Ingredients:
- 3 slices whole grain bread (ensure it's freshly baked to avoid preservatives)
- 1 ripe avocado
- 1 tbsp lemon juice
- Salt and pepper to taste
- 1 cup mixed berries

Instructions:
1. Toast the bread slices until golden brown.
2. Mash the avocado with lemon juice, salt, and pepper.
3. Spread the mashed avocado on each slice of toast.
4. Serve with a side of mixed berries.

Nutritional Info (per serving):

- Calories: 220
- Protein: 5g
- Fat: 15g
- Carbs: 25g
- Fiber: 9g
- Iron: 1.5mg

Tips:

- Choose freshly baked or homemade whole grain bread to avoid preservatives that could trigger histamine reactions.
- Avocados and berries are both nutrient-rich and generally safe for a low-histamine diet.

General Tips for a Low-Histamine Diet:

- Avoid foods that are aged, fermented, or preserved, such as aged cheeses, cured meats, and pickled vegetables, as they tend to have higher histamine levels.

- Focus on fresh, whole ingredients, and cook meals from scratch to control histamine intake.
- Work with a dietitian to customize your meals based on your personal histamine tolerance.

These meals are crafted to support your health while keeping histamine levels low. By using fresh, whole foods and incorporating fiber, healthy fats, and antioxidants, you can maintain balance while enjoying a satisfying diet. Keep meals varied and nutrient-dense to promote overall well-being.

6. Kale, Apple, and Almond Milk Smoothie

Preparation Time:

- 5 minutes
- Serves: 2

Ingredients:

- 1 cup fresh kale, chopped
- 1 medium apple (peeled and cored)
- 1 cup unsweetened almond milk
- 1 tablespoon chia seeds
- 1 teaspoon lemon juice
- 1/2 teaspoon cinnamon (optional)
- 1-2 ice cubes (optional)

Directions:

1. Place the kale, apple, almond milk, chia seeds, and lemon juice in a blender.
2. Blend until smooth, adding ice cubes for extra chill, if preferred.
3. Pour into glasses and enjoy immediately.

<u>**Nutritional Information (per serving):**</u>

- Calories: 90
- Protein: 2g
- Carbs: 22g
- Fiber: 4g
- Fat: 3g
- Vitamin C: 15% of daily value
- Calcium: 15% of daily value

Tips:

- Use tart apples like Granny Smith to enhance the kale flavor.
- Almond milk is a great option, as it is low in histamine and promotes iron absorption.

7. Banana and Nut Butter Smoothie

Preparation Time:
- 5 minutes
- Serves: 1

Ingredients:
- 1 ripe banana
- 1 tablespoon almond butter (or unsweetened peanut butter)
- 1 cup unsweetened almond milk
- 1/2 teaspoon cinnamon
- 1/2 teaspoon vanilla extract (optional)
- 1 tablespoon flax seeds (optional)

Directions:
1. Combine all ingredients in a blender and blend until smooth.
2. Pour into a glass and serve immediately.

Nutritional Information (per serving):

- Calories: 230
- Protein: 6g
- Carbs: 30g
- Fiber: 5g
- Fat: 12g
- Potassium: 450mg
- Vitamin E: 10% of daily value

Tips:

- Freeze the banana beforehand for a thicker smoothie texture.
- Nut butters offer healthy fats and protein, with almond butter being particularly suitable for a low histamine diet.

8. Chia Pudding with Blueberries (Overnight)

Preparation Time:

- 10 minutes
- (plus 4 hours or overnight to set)
- Serves: 2

Ingredients:

- 3 tablespoons chia seeds
- 1 cup unsweetened almond milk
- 1/2 teaspoon vanilla extract
- 1/2 teaspoon cinnamon (optional)
- 1/4 cup fresh or frozen blueberries
- 1 teaspoon maple syrup (optional)

Directions:

1. Mix chia seeds, almond milk, vanilla extract, and cinnamon in a bowl or jar.

2. Stir well and refrigerate overnight or for at least 4 hours.

3. Top with blueberries and drizzle with maple syrup just before serving.

Nutritional Information (per serving):

- Calories: 120
- Protein: 4g
- Carbs: 14g
- Fiber: 10g
- Fat: 7g
- Antioxidants: High in antioxidants from chia seeds and blueberries

Tips:

- Chia seeds are an excellent source of omega-3 fatty acids.
- Adjust the sweetness by adding maple syrup or a stevia substitute to suit your taste.

9. Sweet Potato Hash with Scrambled Eggs

Preparation Time:

- 20 minutes
- Serves: 2

Ingredients:

- 2 medium sweet potatoes, peeled and diced
- 1 tablespoon olive oil
- 1/2 bell pepper, chopped
- 1/4 red onion, chopped
- 2 large eggs
- Salt and pepper, to taste
- Fresh parsley (optional, for garnish)

Directions:

1. Heat olive oil in a skillet over medium heat.
2. Add sweet potatoes and cook for 10 minutes, stirring occasionally, until tender.
3. Add bell pepper and onion, and cook for another 5 minutes.

4. Meanwhile, whisk eggs with salt and pepper.

5. Scramble the eggs in a separate pan or in the same skillet after the veggies are ready.

6. Mix the scrambled eggs with the sweet potato hash and garnish with parsley.

Nutritional Information (per serving):

- Calories: 280
- Protein: 8g
- Carbs: 33g
- Fiber: 6g
- Fat: 14g
- Vitamin A: 150% of daily value (from sweet potatoes)

Tips:

- Sweet potatoes are a great source of complex carbohydrates and antioxidants.
- For a lighter option, use egg whites instead of whole eggs.

10. Cinnamon-Spiced Apple Compote with Cottage Cheese

Preparation Time:

- 15 minutes
- Serves: 6

Ingredients:

- 4 medium apples (peeled, cored, and chopped)
- 1 tablespoon cinnamon
- 1 teaspoon ground ginger
- 1 tablespoon honey (optional)
- 1 tablespoon lemon juice
- 1/2 cup water
- 2 cups low-fat cottage cheese (unsweetened)

Directions:

1. In a saucepan, combine apples, cinnamon, ginger, honey, and lemon juice.
2. Add water and cook over medium heat for 8-10 minutes, stirring occasionally, until apples soften.
3. Once softened, remove from heat and let cool slightly.
4. Spoon cottage cheese into bowls and top with the apple compote.
5. Serve and enjoy!

Nutritional Information (per serving):

- Calories: 120
- Protein: 10g
- Carbs: 20g
- Fiber: 3g
- Fat: 4g

- Limit honey or sweeteners to avoid histamine release.
- Opt for apples with a lower glycemic index, such as Fuji or Gala.

11. Mango and Coconut Chia Smoothie

Preparation Time:
- 5 minutes
- Serves: 6

Ingredients:
- 2 ripe mangoes (peeled and chopped)
- 1/2 cup unsweetened coconut milk (or another plant-based milk)
- 1 tablespoon chia seeds
- 1/2 cup ice cubes
- 1 tablespoon lime juice
- 1 teaspoon vanilla extract (optional)

Directions:

1. Combine mangoes, coconut milk, chia seeds, ice cubes, lime juice, and vanilla extract in a blender.
2. Blend until smooth and creamy.
3. Adjust the sweetness as desired, then pour into glasses and serve immediately.

Nutritional Information (per serving):

- Calories: 110
- Protein: 2g
- Carbohydrates: 23g
- Fiber: 5g
- Fat: 3g

Tips:

- Use unsweetened coconut milk to keep the sugar content low.
- Mangoes are high in vitamin C, which can aid in iron absorption from plant-based foods.

12. Mushroom and Avocado Breakfast Tacos

Preparation Time:
- 15 minutes
- Serves: 6

Ingredients:
- 6 small corn tortillas (choose corn to reduce gluten)
- 1 cup mushrooms (sliced, such as cremini or button)
- 1 ripe avocado (sliced)
- 1/2 cup diced tomatoes
- 1/4 cup fresh cilantro (chopped)
- 2 tablespoons olive oil
- 1/2 teaspoon ground cumin
- Salt and pepper to taste
- Lime wedges for garnish

MooDirections:

1. Heat olive oil in a skillet over medium heat.

2. Add sliced mushrooms, cumin, salt, and pepper, and sauté for about 5 minutes, until mushrooms are tender.

3. Warm the corn tortillas in a dry skillet or microwave for a few seconds.

4. Once the mushrooms are cooked, spoon them onto the tortillas.

5. Top with avocado, tomatoes, and cilantro.

6. Serve with lime wedges for added zest.

Nutritional Information (per serving):

- Calories: 150
- Protein: 3g
- Carbs: 18g
- Fiber: 6g
- Fat: 9g

- Use corn tortillas to minimize processed ingredients.
- Avocados are rich in healthy fats and fiber, making them a great addition to a low histamine diet.
- Mushrooms are low in histamine and rich in antioxidants, making them suitable for this diet.

Chapter 2

Lunches for Maintaining a Low-Histamine Diet

This chapter focuses on creating lunches that help maintain a balanced, low-histamine diet. The meals we will prepare are designed to regulate histamine levels while ensuring you get the essential nutrients for overall health. By choosing ingredients that are either naturally low in histamine or help minimize its impact, we can create flavorful and nourishing lunch options. These meals will incorporate a variety of vegetables, lean proteins, whole grains, and vitamin-rich foods to maintain balance without compromising taste or nutrition. Our approach emphasizes moderation and mindful food choices to support digestive health and energy,

while steering clear of high-histamine
foods.

1. Chickpea Salad with Lemon-Tahini Dressing

Preparation Time:
- 15 minutes
- Serves: 2

Ingredients:
- 1 cup canned chickpeas, rinsed and drained
- 1 cucumber, chopped
- 1 medium tomato, chopped
- 1/2 red onion, thinly sliced
- 1/4 cup fresh parsley, chopped
- 1 tbsp olive oil
- 1 tbsp tahini
- 1 tbsp fresh lemon juice
- 1 tsp ground cumin
- Salt and pepper to taste

Instructions:

1. In a large bowl, combine chickpeas, cucumber, tomato, onion, and parsley.
2. In a separate bowl, mix olive oil, tahini, lemon juice, cumin, salt, and pepper.
3. Pour the dressing over the salad and toss well.
4. Serve immediately or refrigerate for a cooler dish.

Nutrition (per serving):

- Calories: 350
- Protein: 12g
- Carbs: 45g
- Fiber: 12g
- Fat: 15g

Tips:

- Pair with a small portion of brown rice or quinoa for added fiber and energy. Avoid high-histamine ingredients like cured meats or aged cheeses.

2. Quinoa and Roasted Vegetable Bowl

Preparation Time:

- 35 minutes
- Serves: 2

Ingredients:

- 1/2 cup quinoa
- 1 zucchini, sliced
- 1 red bell pepper, sliced
- 1 sweet potato, diced
- 1 tbsp olive oil
- 1 tsp dried oregano
- 1/2 tsp turmeric
- Salt and pepper to taste
- 1 tbsp lemon juice
- 1/4 cup fresh cilantro, chopped

Instructions:

1. Preheat the oven to 400°F (200°C) and line a baking sheet with parchment paper.
2. Toss zucchini, bell pepper, and sweet potato with olive oil, oregano, turmeric, salt, and pepper.
3. Roast for 25-30 minutes, stirring halfway, until vegetables are tender.
4. Cook quinoa according to package instructions.
5. Combine the quinoa with the roasted vegetables, drizzle with lemon juice, and sprinkle with cilantro.

Nutrition (per serving):

- Calories: 350
- Protein: 9g
- Carbs: 60g
- Fiber: 8g
- Fat: 10g

- Add protein by topping with pumpkin or sunflower seeds. Make sure to avoid high-histamine foods like tomatoes or fermented items to keep it low histamine.

3. Grilled Chicken Salad with Mixed Greens

Preparation Time:
- 25 minutes
- Serves: 2

Ingredients:
- 2 boneless, skinless chicken breasts
- 4 cups mixed greens (spinach, arugula, lettuce)
- 1/2 cucumber, sliced
- 1/2 avocado, sliced
- 1/4 cup cherry tomatoes, halved
- 1 tbsp olive oil
- 1 tbsp apple cider vinegar
- 1 tsp Dijon mustard

- Salt and pepper to taste

Instructions:

1. Heat the grill or grill pan to medium-high.
2. Rub the chicken breasts with olive oil, salt, and pepper.
3. Grill for 6-7 minutes per side, or until the internal temperature reaches 165°F (74°C).
4. While the chicken cooks, arrange mixed greens, cucumber, avocado, and cherry tomatoes on plates.
5. Whisk together apple cider vinegar, Dijon mustard, salt, and pepper.
6. Slice the grilled chicken and add on top of the salad, drizzling the dressing over it.

Nutrition (per serving):

- Calories: 300
- Protein: 35g
- Carbs: 10g
- Fiber: 6g
- Fat: 15g

- To avoid histamine, choose fresh chicken over aged or processed options. Limit spinach if you're sensitive to oxalates.

4. Lentil Soup with Carrots and Celery

Preparation Time:

- 40 minutes
- Serves: 2

Ingredients:

- 1/2 cup dried lentils, rinsed
- 1 large carrot, diced
- 2 celery stalks, chopped
- 1/2 onion, chopped
- 1 garlic clove, minced
- 4 cups low-sodium vegetable broth
- 1 tbsp olive oil
- 1 tsp ground cumin
- 1/2 tsp ground turmeric
- Salt and pepper to taste

- 1 tbsp fresh parsley, chopped (for garnish)

Instructions:

1. Heat olive oil in a large pot over medium heat.
2. Add onion, garlic, carrot, and celery and sauté for 5-7 minutes until softened.
3. Stir in cumin, turmeric, salt, pepper, and lentils.
4. Pour in vegetable broth, bring to a boil, then reduce heat and simmer for 25-30 minutes until lentils are tender.
5. Serve with a garnish of fresh parsley.

Nutrition (per serving):

- Calories: 280
- Protein: 18g
- Carbs: 45g
- Fiber: 12g
- Fat: 7g

- Choose low-histamine vegetable broths and avoid adding fermented or pickled ingredients to keep the dish compliant with a low histamine diet.

5. Avocado and Cucumber Rice Paper Rolls

Preparation Time:
- 20 minutes
- Serves: 6

Ingredients:
- 12 rice paper sheets
- 1 ripe avocado, sliced
- 1 cucumber, thinly sliced
- 1 cup shredded carrots
- 1 cup lettuce (romaine or butterhead), chopped
- Fresh cilantro, a handful
- 1 tbsp sesame seeds (optional)
- Low-sodium soy sauce for dipping

- Rice vinegar (optional, for dipping sauce)

Instructions:

1. Prepare the vegetables by julienning the cucumber, slicing the avocado, and shredding the carrots.

2. Soften each rice paper sheet by dipping it into warm water for 10-15 seconds.

3. Lay the softened rice paper on a clean, damp towel or cutting board.

4. Place slices of avocado, cucumber, shredded carrots, and lettuce in the center. Optionally add cilantro and sesame seeds.

5. Fold the sides inward and roll tightly from the bottom.

6. Repeat with the remaining sheets and serve with low-sodium soy sauce or rice vinegar.

Nutrition (per roll):

- Calories: 100 kcal
- Protein: 2g
- Carbohydrates: 15g
- Fiber: 4g

- Fat: 5g

- To keep this dish low in histamine, avoid fermented soy sauces or other aged ingredients, and opt for fresh herbs and vegetables.

6. Spinach and Feta Stuffed Chicken Breast

Preparation Time:

- 35 minutes
- Serves: 6

Ingredients:

- 6 boneless, skinless chicken breasts
- 1 cup fresh spinach (avoid using frozen spinach to prevent higher histamine levels)
- 1/2 cup feta cheese (freshly made, not aged)
- 1 tablespoon olive oil

- 1 teaspoon garlic powder
- 1 teaspoon onion powder
- Salt and pepper to taste

Instructions:

1. Preheat the oven to 375°F (190°C).

2. Heat olive oil in a pan over medium heat and cook fresh spinach until wilted.

3. Combine spinach with feta cheese, garlic powder, onion powder, salt, and pepper.

4. Cut a small pocket in each chicken breast and stuff with the spinach and feta mixture.

5. Secure the chicken breasts with toothpicks and season with salt and pepper.

6. Place the chicken in a baking dish and bake for 25-30 minutes, or until fully cooked (internal temperature of 165°F/74°C).

7. Serve immediately.

<u>Nutritional Information (per serving):</u>

- Calories: 240 kcal
- Protein: 30g
- Carbohydrates: 3g
- Fiber: 1g
- Fat: 12g

Tips:

- Choose freshly made feta cheese and avoid aged versions to minimize histamine content.
- Serve with roasted vegetables like zucchini or carrots for a balanced meal.

7. Roasted Sweet Potato and Black Bean Tacos

Preparation Time:
- 40 minutes
- Serves: 6

Ingredients:
- 3 medium sweet potatoes, peeled and cubed
- 1 can black beans, drained and rinsed
- 1 tablespoon olive oil
- 1 teaspoon cumin
- 1 teaspoon smoked paprika (ensure it's fresh)
- Salt and pepper to taste
- 6 small corn tortillas
- 1/2 cup chopped red onion
- 1/2 cup fresh cilantro, chopped
- Lime wedges for serving
- Avocado slices (optional)

Instructions:

1. Preheat the oven to 400°F (200°C).

2. Toss sweet potato cubes with olive oil, cumin, smoked paprika, salt, and pepper. Spread evenly on a baking sheet.

3. Roast for 25-30 minutes until soft and lightly caramelized.

4. While the sweet potatoes are roasting, heat the black beans over medium heat for 5-7 minutes.

5. Warm the corn tortillas in a dry skillet or oven.

6. Assemble tacos by adding sweet potatoes and black beans to each tortilla, then topping with red onion, cilantro, and optional avocado slices.

7. Serve with lime wedges.

Nutritional Information (per taco):

- Calories: 180 kcal
- Protein: 6g
- Carbohydrates: 35g
- Fiber: 7g

- Fat: 3g

- Use freshly prepared black beans, as canned beans may have preservatives.
- Ensure no aged cheese or fermented products are added.
- Pair with a side of mixed greens for extra nutrients.

8. Turkey Lettuce Wraps with Avocado

Preparation Time:

- 25 minutes
- Serves: 6

Ingredients:

- 1 lb ground turkey (lean, skinless)
- 1 tablespoon olive oil
- 1 teaspoon garlic powder
- 1 teaspoon onion powder

- 1/2 teaspoon paprika
- 1 tablespoon low-sodium soy sauce (check for additives)
- 1 tablespoon rice vinegar (fresh, not aged)
- 1 avocado, diced
- 1 small cucumber, thinly sliced
- 12 large lettuce leaves (such as butter or iceberg lettuce)

Instructions:

1. Heat olive oil in a large skillet over medium heat. Add ground turkey, garlic powder, onion powder, paprika, and soy sauce. Cook until browned (7-10 minutes).

2. Stir in rice vinegar and remove from heat.

3. Wash and dry the lettuce leaves.

4. To assemble, place a spoonful of turkey mixture in each lettuce leaf.

5. Top with diced avocado and cucumber slices.

6. Serve immediately.

Nutritional Information (per wrap):

- Calories: 150 kcal
- Protein: 20g
- Carbohydrates: 4g
- Fiber: 3g
- Fat: 8g

Tips:

- Use freshly cooked ground turkey to avoid histamine buildup.
- Avoid adding fermented sauces or pre-prepared soy sauce.
- For a meat-free alternative, swap turkey for lentils or tofu, and ensure they're freshly prepared.

9. Grilled Shrimp Salad with Mango Salsa

Preparation Time:

- 25 minutes
- Serves: 4

Ingredients:

- 1 lb shrimp, peeled and deveined
- 1 mango, diced
- 1 cup mixed greens (such as spinach or kale)
- 1 tablespoon olive oil
- Juice from 1 lime
- Salt and pepper to taste

Instructions:

1. Heat the grill or grill pan to medium.

2. Toss the shrimp in olive oil, salt, and pepper. Grill for 2-3 minutes per side until fully cooked.

3. Mix diced mango, lime juice, salt, and pepper to make salsa.

4. Arrange the mixed greens on plates and place grilled shrimp on top.

5. Spoon over the mango salsa and serve immediately.

Nutritional Information (per serving):

- Calories: 250
- Protein: 25g
- Carbohydrates: 15g
- Fiber: 4g
- Fat: 12g

Tips:

- Choose sustainably sourced, fresh shrimp to minimize histamine levels.
- Mango's vitamin C aids absorption of iron, making it a great addition to meals.

10. Zucchini Noodles with Pesto and Cherry Tomatoes

Preparation Time:
- 20 minutes
- Serves: 4

Ingredients:
- 4 medium zucchinis, spiralized into noodles
- 1 cup fresh basil leaves
- 1/4 cup pine nuts
- 2 tablespoons olive oil
- 1/2 cup cherry tomatoes, halved
- 1 tablespoon nutritional yeast (optional, ensure it's fresh)

Instructions:
1. Blend basil, pine nuts, olive oil, and nutritional yeast (if using) in a food processor until smooth.

2. Heat a large pan over medium heat and sauté zucchini noodles for 2-3 minutes until tender.

3. Stir in pesto and toss to coat noodles.

4. Add halved cherry tomatoes and toss again.

5. Serve immediately with extra basil if desired.

Nutritional Information (per serving):

- Calories: 220
- Protein: 6g
- Carbohydrates: 16g
- Fiber: 5g
- Fat: 18g

Tips:

- Use freshly prepared pesto without aged cheese for a suitable version.
- Zucchini noodles are a, nutritious alternative to pasta.

11. Mediterranean Hummus and Veggie Wrap

Preparation Time:
- 15 minutes
- Serves: 4

Ingredients:
- 4 whole wheat wraps or tortillas
- 1 cup hummus (preferably homemade or low-sodium)
- 1 cup cucumber, sliced
- 1/2 cup red bell pepper, sliced
- 1/4 cup Kalamata olives, chopped
- 1 tablespoon olive oil
- Fresh parsley for garnish

Instructions:
1. Lay the wraps flat.
2. Spread 1/4 cup of hummus on each wrap.
3. Layer with cucumber, bell pepper, and olives.
4. Drizzle with olive oil and sprinkle with fresh parsley.

5. Roll wraps tightly and cut in half for easy serving.

Nutritional Information (per serving):

- Calories: 300
- Protein: 8g
- Carbohydrates: 30g
- Fiber: 8g
- Fat: 16g

Tips:

- Opt for homemade or freshly made hummus to avoid additives and preservatives.
- Pair with fresh veggies to enhance the meal's nutrient content.

12. Cauliflower Rice and Chickpea Stir Fry

Preparation Time:

- 30 minutes
- Serves: 4

Ingredients:

- 1 medium cauliflower, grated into rice-sized pieces
- 1 can chickpeas, drained and rinsed
- 1 tablespoon olive oil
- 1/2 onion, diced
- 1 cup bell peppers, diced
- 1 tablespoon low-sodium soy sauce (check ingredients for additives)
- 1/2 teaspoon ground turmeric
- 1/2 teaspoon cumin
- Fresh cilantro for garnish

Instructions:

1. Pulse cauliflower in a food processor until it resembles rice.

2. Heat olive oil in a pan over medium heat. Add diced onion and cook for 3-4 minutes.

3. Add bell peppers and cook for another 3 minutes.

4. Stir in chickpeas, turmeric, cumin, and soy sauce, cooking for 5 minutes.

5. Add cauliflower rice, stir, and cook for another 5-7 minutes.

6. Garnish with cilantro before serving.

Nutritional Information (per serving):

- Calories: 200
- Protein: 10g
- Carbohydrates: 30g
- Fiber: 8g
- Fat: 8g

- Freshly prepared cauliflower rice is a great alternative for a lighter meal.
- Add extra vegetables like spinach or zucchini for more nutrition.

Chapter 3

Low Histamine-Friendly Dinner Ideas

In this chapter, we'll delve into a variety of tasty and nutritious dinner options designed to align with a low histamine diet. The meals provided are carefully crafted to offer well-rounded nutrition while keeping histamine levels in check. By choosing ingredients that are naturally low in histamine and help prevent its accumulation, we can prepare dishes that are both delicious and beneficial for overall well-being. By making mindful selections of protein sources, vegetables, and grains, we'll create meals that promote a healthy balance in the body. Join us as we explore satisfying recipes tailored for a low histamine lifestyle.

1. Grilled Salmon with Steamed Broccoli

Preparation Time:
- 20 minutes
- Serves: 2

Ingredients:
- 2 fresh salmon fillets (4-6 oz each)
- 1 tablespoon olive oil
- 1 tablespoon lemon juice
- Salt and pepper to taste
- 1 cup broccoli florets
- 1 teaspoon garlic powder (optional)

Instructions:
1. Preheat the grill or grill pan to medium-high.
2. Coat the salmon with olive oil, lemon juice, salt, and pepper.
3. Grill the salmon for 4-6 minutes per side, or until fully cooked and flakes easily.

4. Steam the broccoli in a steamer basket for 5-7 minutes, seasoning with salt, pepper, and garlic powder.

5. Serve the salmon with the broccoli.

Nutritional Value (per serving):

- Calories: 380
- Protein: 38g
- Fat: 24g
- Carbs: 6g
- Fiber: 3g
- Iron: Low

Tips:

- Use fresh, wild-caught salmon to ensure it's at its freshest and least likely to contain higher histamine levels.
- Broccoli is a great vegetable that is easily digestible and supports overall well-being.

2. Lemon Herb Roasted Chicken with Brussels Sprouts

Preparation Time:
- 35 minutes
- Serves: 2

Ingredients:
- 2 skinless, boneless chicken breasts
- 1 tablespoon olive oil
- 1 tablespoon lemon zest
- 1 tablespoon fresh thyme or rosemary (or 1 teaspoon dried)
- Salt and pepper to taste
- 1 cup Brussels sprouts, halved
- 1 teaspoon garlic powder

Instructions:
1. Preheat the oven to 375°F (190°C).
2. Rub the chicken with olive oil, lemon zest, thyme (or rosemary), salt, and pepper.
3. Roast the chicken on a baking sheet for 25-30 minutes, or until the internal temperature reaches 165°F (74°C).

4. Toss the Brussels sprouts with olive oil, salt, pepper, and garlic powder, then roast them for 20-25 minutes until golden and tender.

5. Serve the chicken alongside Brussels sprouts.

Nutritional Value (per serving):

- Calories: 320
- Protein: 42g
- Fat: 14g
- Carbs: 10g
- Fiber: 4g
- Iron: Low

Tips:

- Fresh chicken is ideal for those with sensitivities, offering lean protein and low histamine content.
- Brussels sprouts are a great option for adding fiber while avoiding high histamine foods.

3. Eggplant and Zucchini Stir-Fry

Preparation Time:

- 20 minutes
- Serves: 2

Ingredients:

- 1 medium eggplant, cubed
- 1 medium zucchini, sliced
- 1 bell pepper, sliced
- 1 tablespoon sesame oil
- 2 tablespoons low-sodium soy sauce (fresh)
- 1 tablespoon rice vinegar
- 1 teaspoon grated ginger
- 1 clove garlic, minced
- 1 tablespoon sesame seeds (optional)

Instructions:

1. Heat sesame oil in a large skillet or wok over medium-high heat.

2. Add garlic and ginger, cooking for 1-2 minutes until fragrant.

3. Add eggplant, zucchini, and bell pepper to the pan, stir-frying for 5-7 minutes until tender.

4. Stir in soy sauce and rice vinegar, cooking for another 2-3 minutes.

5. Sprinkle sesame seeds on top before serving.

Nutritional Value (per serving):

- Calories: 150
- Protein: 3g
- Fat: 8g
- Carbs: 18g
- Fiber: 6g
- Iron: Low

Tips:

- This vegetable stir-fry provides a flavorful, light meal without adding histamine.
- Bell peppers and other fresh vegetables help enhance nutrient absorption while being gentle on digestion.

4. Beef Stir-Fry with Bell Peppers and Broccoli

Preparation Time:
- 25 minutes
- Serves: 2

Ingredients:
- 6 oz lean beef (e.g., sirloin, fresh, not aged), thinly sliced
- 1 tablespoon olive oil
- 1 red bell pepper, sliced
- 1 cup broccoli florets
- 2 tablespoons low-sodium soy sauce (fresh)
- 1 tablespoon oyster sauce (optional, ensure it's fresh)
- 1 tablespoon minced garlic
- 1 teaspoon fresh ginger, minced

Instructions:
1. Heat olive oil in a wok or large skillet over medium-high heat.
2. Add garlic and ginger, sautéing for 1 minute.

3. Add the beef slices, stir-frying for 2-3 minutes until browned.

4. Add the bell pepper and broccoli, stir-frying for another 3-4 minutes until tender.

5. Stir in soy sauce and oyster sauce, cooking for another 1-2 minutes.

6. Serve the stir-fry over brown rice or quinoa for a complete meal.

Nutritional Value (per serving):

- Calories: 350
- Protein: 35g
- Fat: 15g
- Carbs: 15g
- Fiber: 5g
- Iron: Moderate (due to beef)

Tips:

- Use fresh, lean beef to minimize any potential histamine build-up.
- Adding more vegetables and reducing the beef portion can help balance the meal and manage sensitivities.

5. Grilled Shrimp with Asparagus and Quinoa

Preparation Time:

- 25 minutes
- Serves: 2

Ingredients:

- 12 large shrimp, peeled and deveined (fresh, not frozen)
- 1 tablespoon olive oil
- 1 teaspoon lemon zest
- Salt and pepper, to taste
- 1 bunch asparagus, trimmed and cut into 2-inch pieces
- 1 cup quinoa
- 2 cups water or low-sodium broth

Instructions:

1. Preheat the grill to medium-high heat.

2. Toss the shrimp with olive oil, lemon zest, salt, and pepper.

3. Grill the shrimp for 2-3 minutes on each side until cooked through.

4. While grilling, bring water or broth to a boil in a saucepan, then add quinoa. Lower heat and simmer for 15 minutes until the liquid is absorbed.

5. Steam the asparagus in a steamer basket for 5-7 minutes until tender.

6. Serve the shrimp over quinoa, with the asparagus on the side.

Nutritional Value (per serving):

- Calories: 400
- Protein: 35g
- Fat: 12g
- Carbs: 40g
- Fiber: 6g
- Iron: Low

Tips:

- Shrimp is a great protein source for those avoiding high histamine foods, offering flavor without added complications.
- Asparagus and quinoa provide fiber and nutrients, supporting digestion while remaining gentle on the body.

- Choose fresh proteins (chicken, fish, shrimp) and avoid aged or preserved meats.
- Incorporate fresh, non-fermented vegetables like broccoli, zucchini, and bell peppers.
- Limit processed and fermented foods, including soy sauce (ensure it's freshly made) or anything aged.
- Increase fiber-rich vegetables like asparagus, bell peppers, and quinoa to enhance digestion.
- Stay hydrated with water or mild teas, and eat a variety of vegetables for a nutrient-packed meal.

6. Spaghetti Squash with Garlic and Olive Oil

Preparation Time:

- 15 minutes
- Cook Time: 45 minutes
- Serves: 3

Ingredients:

- 1 medium spaghetti squash
- 3 tbsp extra virgin olive oil
- 3 garlic cloves, minced
- Salt and pepper to taste
- 2 tbsp fresh parsley, chopped (optional)
- 1 tbsp lemon zest (optional)

Instructions:

1. Preheat the oven to 400°F (200°C). Cut the spaghetti squash in half lengthwise and remove the seeds.

2. Drizzle 1 tbsp olive oil over the squash and season with salt and pepper. Place the squash cut-side down on a baking sheet.

3. Roast for 40-45 minutes until tender and easily shredded with a fork.

4. While the squash roasts, heat the remaining olive oil in a pan over medium heat. Sauté the garlic for 2-3 minutes until fragrant.

5. Once the squash is done, use a fork to scrape the strands into a bowl and toss with the garlic and olive oil mixture.

6. Garnish with parsley and lemon zest if desired.

Nutritional Information (per serving):

- Calories: 120 kcal
- Protein: 2g
- Carbs: 10g
- Fat: 9g (from olive oil)
- Fiber: 2g

Tips:

- Spaghetti squash serves as a light, pasta alternative. Avoid pairing with high-histamine foods like aged cheeses or fermented items. Enhance with safe vegetables like zucchini or bell peppers.

7. Tofu and Vegetable Curry with Coconut Milk

Preparation Time:

- 15 minutes
- Cook Time: 25 minutes
- Serves: 3

Ingredients:

- 1 block firm tofu, drained and cubed
- 1 tbsp coconut oil
- 1 onion, diced
- 1 bell pepper, chopped
- 1 zucchini, chopped
- 1 carrot, peeled and sliced
- 1 can (14 oz) coconut milk (full-fat)
- 1 tbsp curry powder
- 1 tsp ground turmeric
- Salt to taste

- Fresh cilantro for garnish

Instructions:

1. Heat coconut oil in a large pan over medium heat. Sauté tofu cubes until golden on all sides, about 7-10 minutes. Remove and set aside.

2. In the same pan, add onion, bell pepper, zucchini, and carrot. Cook for 5 minutes until softened.

3. Stir in curry powder, turmeric, and salt. Cook for 1-2 minutes.

4. Add coconut milk and simmer. Return tofu to the pan and cook for 5-10 minutes until the curry thickens and vegetables are tender.

5. Garnish with fresh cilantro before serving.

Nutritional Information (per serving):

- Calories: 250 kcal
- Protein: 15g
- Carbs: 20g
- Fat: 15g (from coconut oil and milk)
- Fiber: 5g

Tips:

- Tofu and coconut milk provide a creamy, plant-based dish without causing histamine issues. Stick to mild vegetables like zucchini and bell peppers for best results.

8. Vegetable and Chickpea Stew

Preparation Time:

- 10 minutes
- Cook Time: 30 minutes
- Serves: 3

Ingredients:

- 1 tbsp olive oil
- 1 onion, diced
- 2 garlic cloves, minced
- 1 carrot, peeled and chopped
- 1 zucchini, chopped
- 1 can (15 oz) chickpeas, drained and rinsed
- 1 can (14 oz) diced tomatoes
- 2 cups vegetable broth (low sodium)
- 1 tsp cumin
- 1 tsp paprika
- Salt and pepper to taste
- Fresh spinach (optional)

Instructions:

1. Heat olive oil in a large pot over medium heat. Add onion and garlic and cook for about 5 minutes.

2. Add carrot and zucchini and cook for another 5 minutes.

3. Stir in chickpeas, tomatoes, vegetable broth, cumin, paprika, salt, and pepper. Bring to a boil.

4. Lower the heat and simmer for 20 minutes, or until vegetables are soft.

5. Add spinach during the last 5 minutes and stir to wilt.

6. Serve hot, optionally garnished with fresh herbs or a squeeze of lemon.

Nutritional Information (per serving):

- Calories: 220 kcal
- Protein: 9g
- Carbs: 35g
- Fat: 7g
- Fiber: 10g

- Chickpeas provide excellent plant-based protein, and this stew is full of digestible vegetables. Avoid triggering ingredients like tomatoes or fermented foods, and pair with rice or quinoa for a complete meal.

9. Zucchini and Bell Pepper Frittata

Preparation Time:

- 10 minutes
- Cook Time: 20 minutes
- Serves: 3

Ingredients:

- 6 large eggs
- 1 tbsp olive oil
- 1 small zucchini, sliced
- 1 bell pepper, chopped
- 1 small onion, diced
- Salt and pepper to taste

- 1/4 cup low-fat cheese (optional)
- Fresh herbs (parsley or basil) for garnish

Instructions:

1. Preheat the oven to 375°F (190°C).

2. Heat olive oil in an oven-safe skillet over medium heat. Add zucchini, bell pepper, and onion. Cook for about 5 minutes.

3. Whisk eggs with salt and pepper in a bowl.

4. Pour the eggs over the vegetables and cook for 2-3 minutes until the edges start to set.

5. Transfer the skillet to the oven and bake for 10-12 minutes, until the center is firm.

6. Garnish with fresh herbs and serve warm.

Nutritional Information (per serving):

- Calories: 180 kcal
- Protein: 12g
- Carbs: 7g
- Fat: 14g
- Fiber: 2g

- Eggs provide high-quality protein, and fresh herbs add flavor without triggering sensitivities. Skip aged cheese or cured meats to maintain a safe meal.

10. Baked Chicken Thighs with Roasted Root Vegetables

Preparation Time:

- 15 minutes
- Cook Time: 45 minutes
- Total Time: 1 hour
- Serves: 4

Ingredients:

- 4 bone-in, skin-on chicken thighs
- 3 medium carrots, peeled and chopped
- 2 medium parsnips, peeled and chopped
- 1 medium sweet potato, peeled and diced
- 2 tbsp olive oil
- 1 tsp dried rosemary
- 1 tsp dried thyme

- Salt and pepper to taste
- 2 garlic cloves, minced
- 1 tbsp fresh lemon juice
- 1 tbsp fresh parsley (optional)

Instructions:

1. Preheat the oven to 400°F (200°C).

2. Toss the carrots, parsnips, and sweet potato with 1 tbsp olive oil, rosemary, thyme, salt, and pepper. Spread evenly on a baking sheet.

3. Coat the chicken thighs with the remaining olive oil, garlic, salt, pepper, and lemon juice.

4. Place the chicken thighs on the sheet with the vegetables, skin-side up.

5. Roast for 40-45 minutes, or until the chicken reaches an internal temperature of 165°F (75°C) and the vegetables are tender.

6. Garnish with fresh parsley before serving.

<u>**Nutritional Information (per serving):**</u>

- Calories: 370
- Protein: 29g
- Carbs: 30g
- Fiber: 6g
- Fat: 16g
- Saturated Fat: 3g
- Sodium: 300mg

Tips:

- Opt for fresh ingredients to avoid potential histamine triggers. Choose skinless chicken thighs and pair with leafy greens for a lighter option. Avoid fermented sauces or cured meats.

11. Grilled Shrimp with Asparagus and Quinoa

Preparation Time:

- 10 minutes
- Cook Time: 15 minutes
- Total Time: 25 minutes
- Serves: 4

Ingredients:

- 1 lb large shrimp, peeled and deveined
- 2 tbsp olive oil
- 2 tsp lemon zest
- 1 tbsp fresh lemon juice
- 2 garlic cloves, minced
- Salt and pepper to taste
- 1 bunch asparagus, trimmed and cut into 2-inch pieces
- 1 cup quinoa, rinsed
- 2 cups low-sodium vegetable broth or water
- Fresh parsley, chopped (for garnish)

Instructions:

1. Cook quinoa: Combine quinoa and vegetable broth in a medium saucepan. Bring to a boil, reduce heat, cover, and cook for 15 minutes. Fluff with a fork.

2. Grill shrimp: Toss shrimp with 1 tbsp olive oil, lemon zest, lemon juice, garlic, salt, and pepper. Grill for 2-3 minutes per side until pink and opaque.

3. Grill asparagus: Toss asparagus with remaining olive oil, salt, and pepper. Grill for 4-5 minutes until tender.

4. Serve: Plate quinoa and top with shrimp and asparagus. Garnish with fresh parsley.

Nutritional Information (per serving):

- Calories: 330
- Protein: 35g
- Carbs: 30g
- Fiber: 5g
- Fat: 12g
- Saturated Fat: 2g

- Sodium: 150mg

- Quinoa complements shrimp and asparagus for a nutritious meal. Use fresh herbs and simple seasonings to avoid additives. Avoid marinades with fermented ingredients.

Chapter 4

Snacks for Effective Histamine Control

In this chapter, you will learn how to prepare snacks that promote general health, especially for those on a low histamine diet. The emphasis will be on creating nutrient-dense, low-histamine snacks that help maintain balanced histamine levels while supporting overall well-being. You will discover how to select the right ingredients, pair foods for better absorption, and create simple, flavorful snacks that fit a mindful eating approach. These snacks are designed to provide sustained energy and assist your body's natural functions, helping you manage histamine levels in a way that is both effective and enjoyable.

1. Apple Slices with Almond Butter

Preparation Time:

- 5 minutes
- Serves: 2

Ingredients:

- 2 medium apples (Gala or Fuji varieties, which are generally easier to tolerate)
- 2 tablespoons unsweetened almond butter
- A dash of cinnamon (optional, depending on individual sensitivity)

Instructions:

1. Core and slice the apples into thin wedges.

2. Spread almond butter on each slice or serve it in a small dish for dipping.

3. Add a sprinkle of cinnamon if desired.

Nutritional Information (per serving):

- Calories: 150
- Protein: 4g
- Carbs: 20g
- Fiber: 4g
- Fat: 9g (healthy fats from almond butter)
- Iron: Low, as almond butter provides limited iron.

Tips:

- Opt for apples that are less likely to cause discomfort, such as Gala or Fuji.
- Choose natural, unsweetened almond butter without added preservatives or oils.

2. Roasted Chickpeas with Spices

Preparation Time:
- 25 minutes
- Serves: 2

Ingredients:
- 1 can (15 oz) chickpeas, drained and rinsed
- 1 tablespoon olive oil
- 1 teaspoon cumin (if well-tolerated)
- 1/2 teaspoon paprika (use cautiously depending on individual tolerance)
- 1/2 teaspoon garlic powder (omit if garlic is a trigger)
- Salt to taste

Instructions:
1. Preheat the oven to 400°F (200°C).
2. Dry the chickpeas with a paper towel.
3. Toss the chickpeas in olive oil and season with cumin, paprika, garlic powder, and salt.

4. Spread them in a single layer on a baking sheet.

5. Roast for 20-25 minutes, stirring halfway through, until crispy.

Nutritional Information (per serving):

- Calories: 170
- Protein: 9g
- Carbs: 27g
- Fiber: 7g
- Fat: 6g (healthy fats from olive oil)
- Iron: Moderate, with spices influencing absorption.

Tips:

- Add turmeric or coriander for additional flavor without causing discomfort.
- Be mindful of salt if monitoring sodium intake.

3. Greek Yogurt with Walnuts and Honey

Preparation Time:
- 5 minutes
- Serves: 2

Ingredients:
- 1 cup unsweetened Greek yogurt (plain, avoid if dairy is a trigger)
- 2 tablespoons chopped walnuts (if tolerated)
- 1 tablespoon honey (optional)

Instructions:
1. Spoon the Greek yogurt into two bowls.
2. Top with chopped walnuts and drizzle with honey, if desired.
3. Stir gently and serve immediately.

<u>**Nutritional Information (per serving):**</u>

- Calories: 150
- Protein: 10g
- Carbs: 14g
- Fiber: 2g
- Fat: 9g (healthy fats from walnuts)
- Iron: Low, as walnuts and yogurt are not significant sources of iron.

Tips:

- Choose unsweetened yogurt to reduce sugar intake and potential discomfort.
- Ensure walnuts are fresh, as older nuts may cause sensitivities.

4. Carrot and Celery Sticks with Hummus

Preparation Time:
- 5 minutes
- Serves: 2

Ingredients:
- 2 medium carrots, peeled and cut into sticks
- 2 celery stalks, cut into sticks
- 1/4 cup hummus (choose homemade or low-sodium store-bought, avoiding garlic if sensitive)

Instructions:
1. Peel and slice the carrots and celery into sticks.
2. Arrange them on a plate and serve with a small dish of hummus for dipping.

Nutritional Information (per serving):

- Calories: 90
- Protein: 3g
- Carbs: 18g
- Fiber: 6g
- Fat: 3g (from hummus)
- Iron: Low, as carrots and celery are low in iron.

Tips:

- Make your own hummus with fresh ingredients to control any unwanted additives.
- If using store-bought hummus, check for ingredients that may be irritants, such as lemon or preservatives.

5. Rice Cakes with Avocado and Tomato

Preparation Time:
- 5 minutes
- Serves: 2

Ingredients:
- 2 plain rice cakes
- 1 ripe avocado
- 1 small tomato, sliced (use cautiously if tomatoes are a trigger)
- A pinch of salt and pepper
- 1 teaspoon olive oil (optional)

Instructions:
1. Toast the rice cakes if preferred.
2. Mash the avocado in a small bowl and spread evenly over each rice cake.
3. Top with tomato slices, season with salt, pepper, and a drizzle of olive oil if desired.

<u>**Nutritional Information (per serving):**</u>

- Calories: 200
- Protein: 3g
- Carbs: 28g
- Fiber: 6g
- Fat: 12g (healthy fats from avocado and olive oil)
- Iron: Low, as rice cakes and avocado provide minimal iron.

Tips:

- Use fresh herbs like basil or parsley for added flavor without discomfort.
- Check the rice cakes for any preservatives or added flavors that could trigger sensitivities.

- When selecting snacks, focus on fresh, minimally processed foods like apples and vegetables.

- Avoid aged or fermented foods (e.g., cheese, vinegar, and soy products), which may be harder to tolerate.

- Be cautious with certain spices like garlic, onion, and paprika, which can be problematic for some individuals.

- Ensure that all snacks contain a balance of healthy fats, protein, and fiber to help maintain energy levels while following this diet.

6. Cucumber and Hummus Wraps

Preparation Time:
- 10 minutes
- Serves: 6

Ingredients:
- 6 whole wheat or gluten-free wraps
- 1 cup hummus (made with ingredients that are gentle on the digestive system)
- 2 medium cucumbers, thinly sliced
- 1 large avocado, sliced
- 1/2 cup shredded carrots
- 1/4 cup fresh parsley, chopped
- 1/2 teaspoon lemon juice
- Salt and pepper to taste

Instructions:

1. Lay the wraps flat on a cleaned surface.

2. Spread a generous amount of hummus in the center of each wrap.

3. Add the cucumber slices, avocado, shredded carrots, and chopped parsley on top of the hummus.

4. Drizzle with lemon juice and season with salt and pepper.

5. Roll up the wraps tightly, folding in the sides as you go.

6. Cut the wraps in half and serve immediately or refrigerate for later.

Nutritional Value (per serving):

- Calories: 180
- Carbohydrates: 22g
- Protein: 5g
- Fat: 9g
- Fiber: 4g
- Iron: Low

- Select whole wheat wraps to increase fiber, but ensure they are made with ingredients that are easy to digest.
- Opt for a low-sodium hummus to avoid excess salt.
- Consider adding spinach or arugula for extra vitamins without causing any digestive discomfort.

7. Hard-Boiled Eggs with Sea Salt

Preparation Time:
- 10 minutes
- Serves: 6

Ingredients:
- 12 large eggs
- Sea salt to taste
- Freshly ground black pepper (optional)
- Fresh herbs such as parsley or chives (optional)

Instructions:

1. Place eggs in a saucepan and cover with cold water by about an inch.

2. Bring the water to a boil over medium-high heat.

3. Once boiling, cover the pot, turn off the heat, and let it sit for 10-12 minutes.

4. After cooking, transfer the eggs to a bowl of ice water to cool for 5 minutes.

5. Peel the eggs and slice them in half or serve whole.

6. Sprinkle it with sea salt and optional black pepper and herbs for added flavor.

Nutritional Value (per serving):

- Calories: 78
- Carbohydrates: 1g
- Protein: 6g
- Fat: 5g
- Fiber: 0g
- Iron: Moderate

- Hard-boiled eggs are an excellent source of protein and healthy fats, but be mindful of portion sizes due to their impact on digestion.
- Pair with calcium-rich foods or tannin-rich beverages (like green tea) to help reduce the absorption of certain minerals.

8. Homemade Granola with Almonds and Seeds

Preparation Time:
- 15 minutes
- Cook Time: 20-25 minutes
- Serves: 6

Ingredients:
- 2 cups old-fashioned rolled oats
- 1/2 cup chopped almonds
- 1/4 cup sunflower seeds
- 1/4 cup pumpkin seeds

- 1/4 cup chia seeds
- 2 tablespoons honey or maple syrup
- 2 tablespoons coconut oil, melted
- 1/2 teaspoon vanilla extract
- 1/2 teaspoon cinnamon
- 1/4 teaspoon sea salt

Instructions:

1. Preheat the oven to 350°F (175°C) and line a baking sheet with parchment paper.

2. In a large bowl, combine oats, almonds, sunflower seeds, pumpkin seeds, and chia seeds.

3. In a separate bowl, mix together honey (or maple syrup), melted coconut oil, vanilla extract, cinnamon, and sea salt.

4. Pour the wet ingredients over the dry mix and stir until everything is evenly coated.

5. Spread the mixture in an even layer on the baking sheet.

6. Bake for 20-25 minutes, stirring halfway through, until the granola turns golden brown and crispy.

7. Remove from the oven and allow it to cool before serving or storing in an airtight container.

Nutritional Value (per serving):

- Calories: 200
- Carbohydrates: 18g
- Protein: 6g
- Fat: 14g
- Fiber: 4g
- Iron: Low

Tips:

- Use raw or unsweetened nuts and seeds to keep the mixture easy on the stomach.
- Store the granola in an airtight container to maintain freshness. It works well as a snack or breakfast, especially when paired with non-dairy yogurt for a lighter option.
- Add dried fruits like cranberries or apricots sparingly for sweetness, but be mindful of portion sizes.

9. Sliced Pear with Goat Cheese

Preparation Time:
- 10 minutes
- Serves: 5

Ingredients:
- 5 ripe pears (Bartlett or Anjou are ideal)
- 5 oz soft, fresh goat cheese
- 1 tbsp honey (optional)
- 1 tbsp fresh thyme or rosemary (optional for garnish)
- Freshly ground black pepper to taste

Instructions:
1. Wash the pears and slice them into thin wedges, discarding the core and seeds.
2. Arrange the slices on a serving platter.
3. Crumble or slice the goat cheese and scatter over the pear slices.
4. If desired, drizzle honey on top and garnish with thyme or rosemary.
5. Season with freshly ground black pepper.

6. Serve immediately or refrigerate for a short time for a chilled option.

Nutritional Value (per serving):
- Calories: 120 kcal
- Carbohydrates: 16g
- Protein: 4g
- Fat: 7g
- Fiber: 4g
- Iron: 0.5 mg
- Calcium: 80 mg

Tips for Best Results:
- Pears are rich in fiber and antioxidants, supporting digestion and general health.
- Goat cheese is generally easier to digest than many other cheeses, making it a gentler choice.
- Adjust the honey amount to suit your taste and reduce sugar intake.

10. Cashews and Dried Apricots

Preparation Time:
- 5 minutes
- Serves: 5

Ingredients:
- 1 cup raw cashews (unsalted)
- 1/2 cup dried apricots (unsweetened, no sulfur)
- 1 tsp ground cinnamon (optional)

Instructions:
1. Combine cashews and dried apricots in a bowl.
2. If desired, sprinkle ground cinnamon on top for added flavor.
3. Serve right away as a snack or store in an airtight container for up to a week.

Nutritional Value (per serving):

- Calories: 170 kcal
- Carbohydrates: 20g
- Protein: 4g
- Fat: 10g
- Fiber: 3g
- Iron: 1.5 mg
- Calcium: 20 mg

Tips for Best Results:

- Cashews provide heart-healthy fats and energy.
- Dried apricots are a good source of fiber and potassium, but should be consumed in moderation.
- If you need to lighten the snack, reduce the apricots and increase cashews or use dried fruits like apples or blueberries, which tend to be gentler on the system.

11. Roasted Almonds with Cacao Nibs

Preparation Time:
- 15 minutes
- Serves: 5

Ingredients:
- 1 cup raw almonds (unsalted)
- 2 tbsp cacao nibs
- 1 tsp cinnamon (optional)
- 1 tbsp olive oil or coconut oil (optional)
- Sea salt to taste (optional)

Instructions:
1. Preheat the oven to 350°F (175°C).
2. Toss almonds with olive oil or coconut oil in a bowl, then spread them evenly on a baking sheet.
3. Roast for 10-12 minutes or until golden and fragrant, stirring halfway through.
4. Let cool for a few minutes before adding cacao nibs.

5. Optionally, season with sea salt or cinnamon.

6. Serve immediately or store in an airtight container for up to a week.

Nutritional Value (per serving):

- Calories: 160 kcal
- Carbohydrates: 9g
- Protein: 5g
- Fat: 14g
- Fiber: 4g
- Iron: 1.0 mg
- Calcium: 80 mg

Tips for Best Results:

- Almonds are rich in magnesium, promoting heart health and relaxation.
- Cacao nibs provide antioxidants but should be consumed in moderation.
- If concerned about digestion, reduce the cacao nibs or increase the proportion of almonds.

Chapter 5

Delicious Desserts for a Low Histamine Diet

Craving something sweet while managing histamine levels is entirely achievable. This chapter presents a variety of desserts carefully crafted to meet the needs of those following a low histamine diet. The focus is on using ingredients that are naturally low in histamine, avoiding aged or fermented foods, and incorporating fresh, gentle alternatives. Whether it's a refreshing fruit sorbet or a velvety dairy-free mousse, these desserts offer a satisfying way to indulge while staying true to your health objectives. They allow you to enjoy a treat without compromising your dietary balance.

1. Almond Flour Brownies

Preparation Time:
- 15 minutes
- Cook Time: 25 minutes
- Total Time: 40 minutes
- Servings: 2

Ingredients:
- 1 cup almond flour
- 1/4 cup unsweetened cocoa powder
- 1/4 cup erythritol (or another low glycemic sweetener)
- 1/2 teaspoon baking powder
- 1/4 teaspoon salt
- 2 large eggs
- 1/4 cup unsweetened almond milk
- 1/4 cup melted coconut oil
- 1 teaspoon vanilla extract

Instructions:

1. Preheat the oven to 350°F (175°C). Grease a small (8x8 inch) baking pan with coconut oil or line with parchment paper.

2. In a medium bowl, mix almond flour, cocoa powder, erythritol, baking powder, and salt.

3. In another bowl, whisk together the eggs, almond milk, melted coconut oil, and vanilla extract.

4. Combine the wet ingredients with the dry ingredients and mix until smooth.

5. Pour the batter into the prepared pan and spread it evenly.

6. Bake for 20-25 minutes, or until a toothpick comes out clean.

7. Let the brownies cool before cutting into squares and serving.

<u>Nutritional Information (per serving):</u>

- Calories: 220
- Carbs: 6g
- Protein: 6g
- Fat: 18g
- Fiber: 2g
- Sugars: 1g

Tips:

- Avoid consuming high-vitamin C foods to limit iron absorption.
- Use high-quality unsweetened cocoa powder for the best flavor with minimal added sugar.

2. Coconut Chia Seed Pudding

<u>Preparation Time:</u>

- 5 minutes
- Chill Time: 3-4 hours
- Total Time: 3-4 hours
- Servings: 2

Ingredients:

- 1/4 cup chia seeds
- 1 cup unsweetened coconut milk
- 1/2 teaspoon vanilla extract
- 1 tablespoon erythritol or monk fruit sweetener (optional)
- 1/4 cup unsweetened shredded coconut (optional)

Instructions:

1. In a small bowl, mix chia seeds, coconut milk, vanilla extract, and sweetener.

2. Stir well to evenly distribute the chia seeds.

3. Cover and refrigerate for at least 3-4 hours, or overnight for best results.

4. Stir before serving to break up any clumps.

5. Top with shredded coconut if desired and enjoy chilling.

<u>**Nutritional Information (per serving):**</u>

- Calories: 170
- Carbs: 12g
- Protein: 4g
- Fat: 14g
- Fiber: 9g
- Sugars: 1g

<u>*Tips:*</u>

- For optimal digestion, enjoy chia pudding with meals to avoid nutrient absorption interference.
- Substitute almond milk for coconut milk for a different taste.

3. Baked Cinnamon Apples with Walnuts

Preparation Time:

- 10 minutes
- Cook Time: 25 minutes
- Total Time: 35 minutes
- Servings: 2

Ingredients:

- 2 medium apples (such as Fuji or Gala)
- 1/4 cup chopped walnuts
- 1/2 teaspoon ground cinnamon
- 1 tablespoon butter or coconut oil
- 1 teaspoon lemon juice
- A pinch of sea salt

Instructions:

1. Preheat the oven to 350°F (175°C).

2. Core and slice the apples into wedges or rings.

3. Arrange apple slices on a baking sheet and sprinkle with cinnamon, sea salt, and lemon juice.

4. Dot the apples with butter or coconut oil.

5. Bake for 20-25 minutes, or until the apples are tender and slightly caramelized.

6. Toast walnuts in a dry pan over medium heat for 3-5 minutes until fragrant.

7. Once the apples are done, top with toasted walnuts and serve.

Nutritional Information (per serving):

- Calories: 180
- Carbs: 22g
- Protein: 2g
- Fat: 12g
- Fiber: 5g
- Sugars: 14g

Tips:

- Apples are high in fiber and antioxidants; combine with protein for a balanced snack.
- Walnuts add healthy fats and a crunchy texture to the dish.

4. Greek Yogurt and Berry Sorbet

Preparation Time:

- 5 minutes
- Freezing Time: 3-4 hours
- Total Time: 3-4 hours
- Servings: 2

Ingredients:

- 1 cup unsweetened Greek yogurt
- 1/2 cup mixed berries (blueberries, raspberries, strawberries)
- 1 tablespoon erythritol or monk fruit sweetener (optional)
- 1 teaspoon lemon juice

Instructions:

1. In a blender or food processor, combine Greek yogurt, mixed berries, sweetener, and lemon juice.
2. Blend until smooth.

3. Pour the mixture into a shallow dish or ice cube trays.

4. Freeze for 3-4 hours or until firm.

5. Once frozen, break into chunks or scoop into bowls and serve.

Nutritional Information (per serving):

- Calories: 150
- Carbs: 10g
- Protein: 15g
- Fat: 7g
- Fiber: 3g
- Sugars: 7g

Tips:

- Choose low-fat Greek yogurt to reduce fat content.
- Avoid consuming with iron-rich foods to minimize potential interactions.

General Diet Tips:

- Focus on plant-based, non-histamine producing sources for improved nutrient absorption.
- Include healthy fats from nuts, seeds, and coconut to support overall wellness.
- Limit processed foods that could trigger histamine responses.

5. Dark Chocolate and Nut Bark

Preparation Time:

- 15 minutes
- Serves: 4

Ingredients:

- 100g dark chocolate (70% cocoa or higher, preferably organic)
- 1/4 cup chopped raw almonds
- 1/4 cup chopped walnuts
- 2 tbsp pumpkin seeds

- 1 tbsp sunflower seeds
- 1/2 tsp sea salt

Instructions:

1. Melt the dark chocolate in a double boiler or microwave, stirring until smooth.
2. Line a baking sheet with parchment paper.
3. Spread the melted chocolate evenly onto the parchment.
4. Sprinkle chopped almonds, walnuts, pumpkin seeds, and sunflower seeds over the chocolate.
5. Add a pinch of sea salt on top.
6. Refrigerate for 1 hour or until firm.
7. Break into pieces and enjoy.

Nutritional Info (per serving):

- Calories: 200
- Protein: 5g
- Fat: 16g
- Carbs: 12g
- Fiber: 3g
- Sugar: 7g

- Opt for high-quality dark chocolate to keep added sugars to a minimum.
- Nuts and seeds provide healthy fats and fiber.

6. Vegan Chocolate Avocado Mousse

Preparation Time:

- 10 minutes
- Serves: 4

Ingredients:

- 1 ripe avocado
- 2 tbsp cocoa powder (ensure it's non-alkalized)
- 2 tbsp maple syrup or agave syrup
- 1/2 tsp vanilla extract (optional, as vanilla may trigger histamine in some people)
- A pinch of salt

Instructions:

1. Scoop out the avocado and place it into a blender or food processor.
2. Add the cocoa powder, maple syrup, vanilla extract (if tolerated), and salt.
3. Blend until smooth and creamy.
4. Adjust sweetness by adding more maple syrup if preferred.
5. Spoon into serving bowls and refrigerate for at least 30 minutes before serving.

Nutritional Info (per serving):

- Calories: 180
- Protein: 2g
- Fat: 14g
- Carbs: 16g
- Fiber: 6g
- Sugar: 7g

- Avocados provide a healthy source of fats, creating a creamy, dairy-free dessert perfect for a low histamine diet.
- Top with fresh, low-histamine fruits such as blueberries for added flavor and antioxidants.

7. Lemon Poppy Seed Muffins

Preparation Time:

- 15 minutes
- Serves: 4

Ingredients:

- 1 cup almond flour
- 1/4 cup coconut flour
- 1/4 cup maple syrup or coconut sugar
- 2 eggs (or flax eggs for a vegan alternative)
- 1/4 cup almond milk (or other plant-based milk that's tolerated)
- 1 tbsp poppy seeds

- Zest of 1 lemon (check tolerance for citrus)
- Juice of 1 lemon
- 1 tsp baking powder
- 1/2 tsp vanilla extract (optional)

Instructions:

1. Preheat the oven to 350°F (175°C).

2. In a mixing bowl, combine the almond flour, coconut flour, baking powder, poppy seeds, and lemon zest.

3. In another bowl, whisk the eggs, maple syrup, almond milk, lemon juice, and vanilla extract (if tolerated).

4. Add the wet ingredients to the dry ingredients and mix until just combined.

5. Spoon the batter into a muffin tin lined with paper liners.

6. Bake for 15–20 minutes, or until a toothpick comes out clean.

7. Let the muffins cool for 10 minutes before serving.

<u>**Nutritional Info (per muffin):**</u>

- Calories: 160
- Protein: 5g
- Fat: 12g
- Carbs: 10g
- Fiber: 3g
- Sugar: 5g

Tips:

- You can substitute oat or coconut milk for almond milk if needed.
- If citrus is a concern, replace the lemon juice with apple cider vinegar (if tolerated) for a tangy flavor.

8. Coconut Flour Cookies with Almonds

Preparation Time:
- 10 minutes
- Serves: 4

Ingredients:
- 1 cup coconut flour
- 1/2 cup unsweetened almond butter
- 2 tbsp maple syrup
- 2 eggs
- 1/2 tsp vanilla extract (optional)
- 1/4 tsp baking soda
- 1/4 cup chopped almonds (ensure nuts are tolerated)

Instructions:
1. Preheat the oven to 350°F (175°C).
2. In a large bowl, mix the coconut flour, baking soda, and chopped almonds.

3. In another bowl, whisk together the almond butter, maple syrup, eggs, and vanilla extract (if tolerated).

4. Combine the wet ingredients with the dry and mix until well combined.

5. Scoop spoonfuls of dough onto a baking sheet lined with parchment paper, pressing them gently into cookie shapes.

6. Bake for 10–12 minutes, or until golden brown.

7. Allow the cookies to cool on a wire rack before serving.

Nutritional Info (per cookie):

- Calories: 150
- Protein: 5g
- Fat: 12g
- Carbs: 8g
- Fiber: 4g
- Sugar: 4g

- For those sensitive to nuts, try swapping almond butter with sunflower seed butter for a low-histamine alternative.
- Store in an airtight container to keep cookies fresh.

9. Chilled Matcha Pudding

Preparation Time:

- 5 minutes
- (plus 2 hours chilling)
- Serves: 4

Ingredients:

- 1 1/2 cups full-fat coconut milk
- 2 tbsp matcha powder (ensure it's low-histamine and high-quality)
- 2 tbsp maple syrup
- 1 tbsp chia seeds (optional for added thickness)
- 1/2 tsp vanilla extract (optional)

<u>Instructions:</u>

1. Blend the coconut milk, matcha powder, maple syrup, and vanilla extract (if tolerated) until smooth.
2. If desired, add chia seeds and blend again.
3. Pour the mixture into small bowls or jars.
4. Refrigerate for at least 2 hours until the pudding thickens and sets.
5. Serve chilled.

<u>Nutritional Info (per serving):</u>

- Calories: 150
- Protein: 2g
- Fat: 12g
- Carbs: 10g
- Fiber: 4g
- Sugar: 7g

Tips:

- Matcha provides antioxidants and a gentle energy boost but always check if it's suitable for your personal tolerance to histamines.

- Add shredded coconut or low-histamine fruits for extra flavor and texture.

10. Strawberry Basil Sorbet

Preparation Time:
- 10 minutes
- (plus freezing time)
- Serves: 4

Ingredients:
- 2 cups fresh strawberries, hulled (ensure they are fresh and not overripe)
- 1/4 cup fresh basil leaves (use fresh basil as older basil may have higher histamine levels)
- 1/4 cup lemon juice (if tolerated)
- 1/4 cup maple syrup
- 1/2 cup water

Instructions:

1. Blend the strawberries, basil, lemon juice (if tolerated), maple syrup, and water in a blender until smooth.
2. Pour the mixture into a shallow dish or ice cream maker.
3. If using a shallow dish, freeze for 2–3 hours, stirring every 30 minutes to avoid ice crystals.
4. Serve immediately after scooping into bowls.

Nutritional Info (per serving):

- Calories: 80
- Protein: 1g
- Fat: 0g
- Carbs: 20g
- Fiber: 4g
- Sugar: 15g

- Make this sorbet in advance and store it in the freezer for up to a week.
- To reduce sugar content, substitute the maple syrup with stevia or agave syrup if tolerated.

Chapter 6

Beverages to Aid in Low Histamine Management

In this chapter, we focus on drinks that help manage low histamine levels, particularly for individuals who need to closely monitor their histamine intake. The beverages covered are chosen to support the body's ability to maintain balanced histamine levels and prevent its accumulation.

Drinks high in vitamin C, like freshly squeezed citrus juices, strawberry smoothies, and fortified plant-based milks, play a vital role in supporting histamine regulation. Herbal teas, such as peppermint and chamomile, are also helpful, promoting digestive health and assisting in controlling histamine levels without causing excessive production.

It is crucial to avoid drinks that may worsen histamine sensitivity, such as coffee, tea, and certain dairy products, as they contain substances that can trigger histamine release or impair its breakdown. Instead, opting for nutrient-dense, low-histamine beverages can help maintain a balanced histamine level and support overall health.

This chapter provides practical advice on creating drinks that not only complement a healthy, low histamine diet but also help regulate histamine levels for long-term well-being.

1. Lemon Ginger Detox Water

Preparation Time:

- 5 minutes
- Serves: 3

Ingredients:

- 1 lemon, sliced
- 1-inch piece of fresh ginger, peeled and sliced
- 3 cups of filtered water
- 1 teaspoon of honey (optional)

Instructions:

1. Slice the lemon and ginger.
2. Place them in a jug.
3. Add water and refrigerate for at least 2 hours.
4. Sweeten with honey if desired.
5. Stir and serve chilled.

<u>**Nutritional Info (per serving):**</u>

- Calories: 8
- Carbs: 2g
- Sugar: 2g
- Vitamin C: 25% of daily value
- Antioxidants: High

Tips:

Ginger supports digestion and reduces inflammation, while lemon boosts vitamin C, which is beneficial for the immune system. Both ingredients are low in histamine. Avoid high-histamine sweeteners like molasses.

2. Green Tea with Mint

Preparation Time:
- 5 minutes
- Serves: 3

Ingredients:
- 3 cups of brewed green tea (cooled)
- A handful of fresh mint leaves
- 1-2 teaspoons of honey (optional)

Instructions:
1. Brew the green tea and cool it.
2. Add fresh mint leaves.
3. Stir in honey if preferred.
4. Chill in the refrigerator for 1 hour and serve.

Nutritional Info (per serving):
- Calories: 2
- Carbs: 0.5g
- Sugar: 0g (if no honey)
- Antioxidants: High (flavonoids)

- Caffeine: Moderate (approx. 25-35 mg per cup)

- Green tea is rich in catechins, which help reduce inflammation. Mint adds flavor and supports digestion. Both ingredients are suitable for a low histamine diet.

3. Turmeric Almond Milk Latte

Preparation Time:
- 7 minutes
- Serves: 3

Ingredients:
- 2 cups of unsweetened almond milk
- 1 teaspoon of ground turmeric
- 1 teaspoon of cinnamon
- 1 teaspoon of honey (optional)
- A pinch of black pepper (to enhance turmeric absorption)

Instructions:

1. Heat almond milk in a saucepan over medium heat.
2. Add turmeric, cinnamon, and black pepper.
3. Whisk until smooth and warmed through.
4. Stir in honey, mix well, and pour into cups.
5. Serve warm.

Nutritional Info (per serving):

- Calories: 40
- Carbs: 3g
- Sugar: 1g
- Protein: 1g
- Healthy fats: 2g (from almond milk)

Tips:

- Turmeric contains curcumin, which has anti-inflammatory effects, making it great for a low histamine diet. Use almond milk without additives, as some may contain histamine-rich ingredients.

4. Berry Infused Iced Tea

Preparation Time:

- 5 minutes
- Serves: 3

Ingredients:

- 3 cups of brewed black tea (cooled)
- 1/2 cup mixed berries (blueberries, strawberries, raspberries)
- 1 tablespoon of lemon juice
- Ice cubes

Instructions:

1. Brew and cool the black tea.

2. In a pitcher, combine the cooled tea, berries, and lemon juice.

3. Refrigerate for 1 hour to let the flavors infuse.

4. Serve over ice.

<u>**Nutritional Info (per serving):**</u>

- Calories: 10
- Carbs: 3g
- Sugar: 2g (from berries)
- Vitamin C: 10% of daily value

Tips:

- Berries are rich in antioxidants and vitamin C, which support immune health and are typically safe in moderate amounts on a low histamine diet. However, black tea should be consumed cautiously as it may not suit everyone on a low histamine plan.

5. Coconut Water and Lime

Preparation Time:
- 3 minutes
- Serves: 3

Ingredients:
- 2 cups of fresh coconut water
- 1 lime, juiced
- 1-2 teaspoons of honey (optional)

Instructions:
1. Mix coconut water with lime juice in a glass.
2. Sweeten with honey if desired.
3. Serve chilled with ice.

Nutritional Info (per serving):
- Calories: 20
- Carbs: 5g
- Sugar: 4g
- Potassium: 10% of daily value

- Coconut water is hydrating and full of electrolytes, making it ideal for staying hydrated. Lime enhances flavor and digestion, both of which are beneficial for a low histamine diet. Choose fresh coconut water without preservatives for the best results.

6. Cucumber and Lemon Infused Water

Preparation Time:
- 5 minutes
- Makes: 3 servings

Ingredients:
- 1 cucumber, sliced
- 1 lemon, sliced
- 4 cups filtered water

Instructions:
1. Thinly slice the cucumber and lemon.
2. Add them to a jug with the water.
3. Let the mixture infuse in the refrigerator for at least 2 hours.
4. Serve chilled with ice cubes.

Nutritional Information (per serving):

- Calories: 5
- Carbs: 1g
- Sugar: 1g
- Vitamin C: 10% of the daily value

Tips:

- This cooling water is ideal for staying hydrated and promoting detoxification. Both cucumber and lemon are gentle on digestion and provide antioxidants that support the body's natural detox processes, making them great choices for a low-histamine diet.

7. Pineapple and Ginger Smoothie

Preparation Time:

- 5 minutes
- Makes: 2 servings

Ingredients:

- 1 cup fresh pineapple chunks
- 1-inch piece fresh ginger, peeled
- 1/2 cup coconut water or regular water
- 1/2 cup ice (optional)
- 1 tablespoon chia seeds (optional for added fiber)

Instructions:

1. Add the pineapple, ginger, and coconut water (or water) to a blender.
2. Blend until smooth.
3. Optionally, include ice and chia seeds for more texture and fiber.
4. Serve immediately.

<u>**Nutritional Information (per serving):**</u>

- Calories: 60 kcal
- Carbs: 15g
- Protein: 0.5g
- Fat: 0.5g
- Fiber: 2g
- Vitamin C: 80% of the daily value

<u>**Tips:**</u>

- Pineapple has bromelain, which helps with digestion, while ginger reduces inflammation. Coconut water is hydrating without adding excess sugar. This smoothie is suitable for a low-histamine diet. Avoid sweeteners to maintain its natural, low-histamine properties.

8. Apple Cider Vinegar and Lemon Drink

Preparation Time:
- 3 minutes
- Makes: 2 servings

Ingredients:
- 1 tablespoon apple cider vinegar (raw, unfiltered)
- Juice of 1/2 lemon
- 2 cups water (filtered or room temperature)
- A pinch of cinnamon (optional)

Instructions:
1. Combine apple cider vinegar, lemon juice, and water in a glass.

2. Stir well and add cinnamon if desired.

3. Serve immediately or store in the fridge for later.

<u>Nutritional Information (per serving):</u>

- Calories: 3 kcal
- Carbs: 1g
- Protein: 0g
- Fat: 0g
- Fiber: 0g
- Vitamin C: 10% of the daily value

Tips:

- Apple cider vinegar aids digestion and detoxification, while lemon contributes vitamin C. This drink supports digestive health and is safe for a low-histamine diet. Limit to two servings daily to avoid any sensitivity.

9. Strawberry Smoothie

Preparation Time:

- 5 minutes
- Makes: 2 servings

Ingredients:

- 1 1/2 cups fresh (or frozen) strawberries
- 1/2 cup unsweetened almond or oat milk
- 1/2 cup spinach (optional for added nutrients)
- 1 teaspoon flax seeds (optional for omega-3s)
- 1/2 banana (optional for sweetness)

Instructions:

1. Blend the strawberries, almond milk, spinach, and flax seeds until smooth.
2. For extra sweetness, add the banana and blend again.
3. Pour into glasses and enjoy!

Nutritional Information (per serving):

- Calories: 45 kcal
- Carbs: 11g
- Protein: 1g
- Fat: 1.5g
- Fiber: 3g
- Vitamin C: 70% of the daily value

Tips:

- Strawberries are rich in antioxidants and vitamin C, which help combat oxidative stress. This smoothie is naturally low in histamine and makes for a delicious, sugar-free treat. Using frozen strawberries can help avoid ice and maintain a smooth consistency.

10. Citrus Juices

Preparation Time:
- 5 minutes
- Makes: 2 servings

Ingredients:
- Juice of 1 orange
- Juice of 1/2 lemon
- 1/2 lime juice
- 1 cup water or sparkling water
- A few mint leaves (optional for garnish)

Instructions:
1. Squeeze the juice from the orange, lemon, and lime into a glass.
2. Add the water or sparkling water and stir well.
3. Garnish with mint leaves if desired.
4. Serve chilled or at room temperature.

<u>**Nutritional Information (per serving):**</u>

- Calories: 40 kcal
- Carbs: 10g
- Protein: 0g
- Fat: 0g
- Fiber: 1g
- Vitamin C: 120% of the daily value

Tips:

- Citrus fruits are packed with vitamin C, which boosts immune health and hydration. Sparkling water gives a refreshing twist, making this juice especially enjoyable in warm weather. This drink is naturally low in histamine and ideal for anyone on a low-histamine diet.

Chapter 7

Living with a Low Histamine Diet Long-Term

Adhering to a low-histamine diet over the long term can be challenging, especially when it comes to staying consistent, maintaining motivation, and ensuring proper nutrition. This chapter offers strategies for thriving with histamine intolerance, including managing social situations, traveling, preventing nutrient deficiencies, and connecting with supportive communities.

Managing a Low Histamine Diet in Social Situations

Attending social events, dining out, or sharing meals with family can feel daunting for someone on a low-histamine diet. However, with preparation, clear communication, and flexibility, these challenges can be overcome.

1. Be Open with Hosts: If you're invited to an event, let your host know about your dietary needs. Many hosts will be happy to accommodate you by preparing dishes that meet your requirements.

2. Bring Your Own Dish: For events like potlucks or barbecues, consider bringing your own food to ensure you have something safe to eat. Simple options like grilled chicken, fresh salads, or quinoa are typically well-received.

3. Dining Out: When eating at a restaurant, it's helpful to call ahead and explain your dietary restrictions. Many restaurants will be willing to prepare meals according to your needs if given advanced notice. When ordering, request dishes made with fresh ingredients and ask about food preparation methods to avoid hidden histamine sources like marinades or processed meats.

4. Educate Friends and Family: Share your dietary restrictions with close friends and family. This can help them understand your needs and make social interactions easier and more supportive.

5. Carry Safe Snacks: Always have low-histamine snacks like fresh fruit, vegetables, or nuts with you. This will help prevent you from reaching for foods that may trigger symptoms.

Traveling with Histamine Intolerance

Traveling while managing histamine intolerance requires careful planning, but it's certainly manageable with the right strategies.

1. Plan Ahead for Meals: Research restaurants, cafes, and grocery stores that can accommodate your dietary needs. Many cities have eateries that cater to health-conscious diners and can offer low-histamine options.

2. Pack Your Own Safe Foods: Bring along travel-friendly snacks like nuts, rice cakes, fresh fruit, or homemade sandwiches. Having your own food will help you avoid making impulsive, potentially harmful choices.

3. Carry Necessary Supplements and Medications: If you rely on antihistamines or supplements to manage your condition, don't forget to pack them. A travel-sized bottle of

DAO (diamine oxidase) can be particularly useful during long trips.

4. Keep Food at the Right Temperature: Histamine levels in food can rise as it warms up. If you're traveling to a hot destination, ensure perishable foods stay cool to prevent histamine buildup.

5. Opt for Accommodations with Kitchens: When booking travel accommodations, choose options with kitchen facilities. This will give you the flexibility to prepare your own meals, ensuring they meet your dietary needs.

Avoiding Nutrient Deficiencies

A restrictive low-histamine diet can sometimes lead to nutrient gaps, but with careful planning, it's possible to maintain a well-balanced diet.

1. Prioritize Whole Foods: Focus on a wide range of fruits, vegetables, grains, and lean proteins. The more variety you incorporate into your meals, the better your chances of meeting all your nutritional requirements.

2. Include Low-Histamine Protein Sources: To support your muscle and immune health, ensure you're consuming enough protein. Opt for low-histamine sources like chicken, turkey, eggs, and tofu.

3. Consider Supplements: If necessary, take supplements to help fill any nutritional gaps. Vitamin C (to support the immune system), magnesium (for muscle and nerve health), and vitamin B6 (which aids in histamine breakdown) are good options to consider.

4. Ensure Balanced Micronutrients: Include a variety of nutrient-dense vegetables like kale, spinach, and broccoli, which will help you meet your vitamin and mineral needs, particularly those that may be depleted on a restricted diet.

5. Consult a Nutritionist: Working with a dietitian who understands histamine intolerance can ensure you're eating in a way that supports both your low-histamine needs and overall health.

Finding Support Groups and Communities

Connecting with others who understand histamine intolerance can make your journey easier. Here are ways to find support:

1. Online Communities: Social media platforms like Facebook and Instagram have numerous groups and hashtags dedicated to histamine intolerance. These communities can offer advice, recipe ideas, and encouragement.

2. Reddit Subreddits: Platforms like Reddit have active subreddits (e.g., r/HistamineIntolerance) where people share experiences, ask questions, and provide helpful tips.

3. In-Person Support Groups: Some areas may offer local support groups for those with histamine intolerance or food sensitivities. Check with health clinics or wellness centers in your area for more information.

4. Specialized Forums: There are various forums dedicated to food sensitivities, where members can discuss diets, share resources, and offer practical advice.

5. Health Coaching or Therapy: If you need emotional or psychological support, consider working with a health coach or therapist who specializes in managing chronic conditions or dietary restrictions.

Staying Motivated: Tips for Long-Term Success

Adhering to a low-histamine diet over time requires persistence and commitment. Here are some tips to help you stay motivated:

1. Set Achievable Goals: Establish both short-term and long-term health goals to help you track your progress. These might include experimenting with new recipes, boosting your energy levels, or reducing flare-ups.

2. Track Symptoms and Improvements: Keep a food journal to identify patterns and figure out which foods work best for you. This can help reinforce your motivation to stick with the diet.

3. Celebrate Small Wins: Recognize and celebrate small achievements, like attending a social event without experiencing symptoms or cooking a new meal that you enjoy. These moments will remind you of the benefits of sticking to the diet.

4. Focus on the Benefits: When you feel tempted to deviate from your low-histamine diet, remind yourself of the long-term benefits, such as improved health, fewer flare-ups, and increased energy.

5. Practice Self-Care: Make time for self-care activities like meditation, exercise, and sleep. These practices will help you stay focused, energized, and emotionally resilient.

30-Day Meal Plan and Shopping List for a Low-Histamine Diet

Creating a 30-day meal plan with low-histamine foods is an excellent strategy for maintaining a balanced, nutrient-dense diet while minimizing histamine intake. This meal plan includes a variety of breakfast, lunch, dinner, snacks, desserts, and beverages that align with low-histamine guidelines. Each day is thoughtfully designed to offer a wide range of flavors and nutrients, ensuring you meet your daily nutritional needs without triggering histamine sensitivity. The plan features diverse, wholesome meals that support overall well-being and adhere to the principles of a low-histamine diet.

Day 1:

- **Breakfast:** Scrambled Eggs with Spinach and Feta
- **Lunch:** Chickpea Salad with Lemon-Tahini Dressing
- **Dinner:** Grilled Chicken Salad with Mixed Greens
- **Snack:** Apple Slices with Almond Butter
- **Dessert:** Almond Flour Brownies
- **Beverage:** Lemon Ginger Detox Water

Day 2:

- **Breakfast:** Oatmeal with Berries and Chia Seeds
- **Lunch:** Quinoa and Roasted Vegetable Bowl
- **Dinner:** Roasted Sweet Potato and Black Bean Tacos
- **Snack:** Greek Yogurt with Walnuts and Honey
- **Dessert:** Coconut Chia Seed Pudding
- **Beverage:** Green Tea with Mint

Day 3:

- **Breakfast:** Greek Yogurt Parfait with Flaxseeds
- **Lunch:** Grilled Shrimp Salad with Mango Salsa
- **Dinner:** Eggplant and Zucchini Stir Fry
- **Snack:** Carrot and Celery Sticks with Hummus
- **Dessert:** Baked Cinnamon Apples with Walnuts

- **Beverage:** Turmeric Almond Milk Latte

Day 4:

- **Breakfast:** Quinoa Porridge with Almond Butter
- **Lunch:** Lentil Soup with Carrots and Celery
- **Dinner:** Zucchini Noodles with Pesto and Cherry Tomatoes
- **Snack:** Roasted Almonds with Cacao Nibs
- **Dessert:** Vegan Chocolate Avocado Mousse
- **Beverage:** Coconut Water and Lime

Day 5:

- **Breakfast:** Avocado Toast with a Side of Berries
- **Lunch:** Mediterranean Hummus and Veggie Wrap
- **Dinner:** Grilled Salmon with Steamed Broccoli

- **Snack:** Hard-Boiled Eggs with Sea Salt
- **Dessert:** Lemon Poppy Seed Muffins
- **Beverage:** Pineapple and Ginger Smoothie

Day 6:

- **Breakfast:** Kale, Apple, and Almond Milk Smoothie
- **Lunch:** Spinach and Feta Stuffed Chicken Breast
- **Dinner:** Tofu and Vegetable Curry with Coconut Milk
- **Snack:** Rice Cakes with Avocado and Tomato
- **Dessert:** Greek Yogurt and Berry Sorbet
- **Beverage:** Cucumber and Lemon Infused Water

Day 7:

- **Breakfast:** Banana and Nut Butter Smoothie
- **Lunch:** Grilled Shrimp with Asparagus and Quinoa
- **Dinner:** Beef Stir-Fry with Bell Peppers and Broccoli
- **Snack:** Cashews and Dried Apricots
- **Dessert:** Strawberry Basil Sorbet
- **Beverage:** Lemon Ginger Detox Water

Day 8:

- **Breakfast:** Chia Pudding with Blueberries (Overnight)
- **Lunch:** Chickpea Salad with Lemon-Tahini Dressing
- **Dinner:** Zucchini and Bell Pepper Frittata
- **Snack:** Greek Yogurt with Walnuts and Honey
- **Dessert:** Dark Chocolate and Nut Bark
- **Beverage:** Coconut Water and Lime

Day 9:

- **Breakfast:** Sweet Potato Hash with Scrambled Eggs
- **Lunch:** Avocado and Cucumber Rice Paper Rolls
- **Dinner:** Grilled Chicken Salad with Mixed Greens
- **Snack:** Sliced Pear with Goat Cheese
- **Dessert:** Almond Flour Brownies
- **Beverage:** Green Tea with Mint

Day 10:

- **Breakfast:** Cinnamon Spiced Apple Compote with Cottage Cheese
- **Lunch:** Quinoa and Roasted Vegetable Bowl
- **Dinner:** Lemon Herb Roasted Chicken with Brussels Sprouts
- **Snack:** Carrot and Celery Sticks with Hummus
- **Dessert:** Chilled Matcha Pudding

- **Beverage:** Apple Cider Vinegar and Lemon Drink

Day 11:

- **Breakfast:** Mushroom and Avocado Breakfast Tacos
- **Lunch:** Grilled Shrimp Salad with Mango Salsa
- **Dinner:** Cauliflower Rice and Chickpea Stir Fry
- **Snack:** Roasted Chickpeas with Spices
- **Dessert:** Coconut Flour Cookies with Almonds
- **Beverage:** Berry Infused Iced Tea

Day 12:

- **Breakfast:** Scrambled Eggs with Spinach and Feta
- **Lunch:** Turkey Lettuce Wraps with Avocado
- **Dinner:** Grilled Shrimp with Asparagus and Quinoa

- **Snack:** Apple Slices with Almond Butter
- **Dessert:** Baked Cinnamon Apples with Walnuts
- **Beverage:** Lemon Ginger Detox Water

Day 13:

- **Breakfast:** Quinoa Porridge with Almond Butter
- **Lunch:** Grilled Chicken Salad with Mixed Greens
- **Dinner:** Vegetable and Chickpea Stew
- **Snack:** Rice Cakes with Avocado and Tomato
- **Dessert:** Vegan Chocolate Avocado Mousse
- **Beverage:** Coconut Water and Lime

Day 14:

- **Breakfast:** Kale, Apple, and Almond Milk Smoothie
- **Lunch:** Mediterranean Hummus and Veggie Wrap

- **Dinner:** Spaghetti Squash with Garlic and Olive Oil
- **Snack:** Greek Yogurt with Walnuts and Honey
- **Dessert:** Coconut Chia Seed Pudding
- **Beverage:** Green Tea with Mint

Day 15:

- **Breakfast:** Oatmeal with Berries and Chia Seeds
- **Lunch:** Quinoa and Roasted Vegetable Bowl
- **Dinner:** Grilled Salmon with Steamed Broccoli
- **Snack:** Cashews and Dried Apricots
- **Dessert:** Strawberry Basil Sorbet
- **Beverage:** Pineapple and Ginger Smoothie

Day 16:

- **Breakfast:** Chia Pudding with Blueberries (Overnight)
- **Lunch:** Chickpea Salad with Lemon-Tahini Dressing
- **Dinner:** Eggplant and Zucchini Stir Fry
- **Snack:** Roasted Almonds with Cacao Nibs
- **Dessert:** Almond Flour Brownies
- **Beverage:** Coconut Water and Lime

Day 17:

- **Breakfast:** Banana and Nut Butter Smoothie
- **Lunch:** Lentil Soup with Carrots and Celery
- **Dinner:** Zucchini Noodles with Pesto and Cherry Tomatoes
- **Snack:** Hard-Boiled Eggs with Sea Salt
- **Dessert:** Greek Yogurt and Berry Sorbet
- **Beverage:** Cucumber and Lemon Infused Water

Day 18:

- **Breakfast:** Avocado Toast with a Side of Berries
- **Lunch:** Quinoa and Roasted Vegetable Bowl
- **Dinner:** Roasted Sweet Potato and Black Bean Tacos
- **Snack:** Apple Slices with Almond Butter
- **Dessert:** Vegan Chocolate Avocado Mousse
- **Beverage:** Green Tea with Mint

Day 19:

- **Breakfast:** Sweet Potato Hash with Scrambled Eggs
- **Lunch:** Grilled Shrimp with Asparagus and Quinoa
- **Dinner:** Grilled Chicken Salad with Mixed Greens
- **Snack:** Carrot and Celery Sticks with Hummus

- **Dessert:** Lemon Poppy Seed Muffins
- **Beverage:** Lemon Ginger Detox Water

Day 20:

- **Breakfast:** Greek Yogurt Parfait with Flaxseeds
- **Lunch:** Avocado and Cucumber Rice Paper Rolls
- **Dinner:** Tofu and Vegetable Curry with Coconut Milk
- **Snack:** Roasted Chickpeas with Spices
- **Dessert:** Dark Chocolate and Nut Bark
- **Beverage:** Coconut Water and Lime

Day 21:

- **Breakfast:** Scrambled Eggs with Spinach and Feta
- **Lunch:** Turkey Lettuce Wraps with Avocado
- **Dinner:** Vegetable and Chickpea Stew
- **Snack:** Sliced Pear with Goat Cheese
- **Dessert:** Almond Flour Brownies

- **Beverage:** Pineapple and Ginger Smoothie

Day 22:

- **Breakfast:** Quinoa Porridge with Almond Butter
- **Lunch:** Grilled Shrimp Salad with Mango Salsa
- **Dinner:** Zucchini and Bell Pepper Frittata
- **Snack:** Cashews and Dried Apricots
- **Dessert:** Strawberry Basil Sorbet
- **Beverage:** Green Tea with Mint

Day 23:

- **Breakfast:** Kale, Apple, and Almond Milk Smoothie
- **Lunch:** Mediterranean Hummus and Veggie Wrap
- **Dinner:** Grilled Salmon with Steamed Broccoli

- **Snack:** Greek Yogurt with Walnuts and Honey
- **Dessert:** Coconut Chia Seed Pudding
- **Beverage:** Lemon Ginger Detox Water

Day 24:

- **Breakfast:** Mango and Coconut Chia Smoothie
- **Lunch:** Quinoa and Roasted Vegetable Bowl
- **Dinner:** Beef Stir-Fry with Bell Peppers and Broccoli
- **Snack:** Rice Cakes with Avocado and Tomato
- **Dessert:** Chilled Matcha Pudding
- **Beverage:** Coconut Water and Lime

Day 25:

- **Breakfast:** Banana and Nut Butter Smoothie
- **Lunch:** Chickpea Salad with Lemon-Tahini Dressing

- **Dinner:** Zucchini Noodles with Pesto and Cherry Tomatoes
- **Snack:** Roasted Almonds with Cacao Nibs
- **Dessert:** Vegan Chocolate Avocado Mousse
- **Beverage:** Berry Infused Iced Tea

Day 26:

- **Breakfast:** Scrambled Eggs with Spinach and Feta
- **Lunch:** Grilled Shrimp Salad with Mango Salsa
- **Dinner:** Eggplant and Zucchini Stir Fry
- **Snack:** Carrot and Celery Sticks with Hummus
- **Dessert:** Almond Flour Brownies
- **Beverage:** Apple Cider Vinegar and Lemon Drink

Day 27:

- **Breakfast:** Oatmeal with Berries and Chia Seeds
- **Lunch:** Avocado and Cucumber Rice Paper Rolls
- **Dinner:** Lemon Herb Roasted Chicken with Brussels Sprouts
- **Snack:** Cashews and Dried Apricots
- **Dessert:** Greek Yogurt and Berry Sorbet
- **Beverage:** Coconut Water and Lime

Day 28:

- **Breakfast:** Chia Pudding with Blueberries (Overnight)
- **Lunch:** Grilled Shrimp with Asparagus and Quinoa
- **Dinner:** Spaghetti Squash with Garlic and Olive Oil
- **Snack:** Apple Slices with Almond Butter
- **Dessert:** Dark Chocolate and Nut Bark
- **Beverage:** Pineapple and Ginger Smoothie

Day 29:

- **Breakfast:** Scrambled Eggs with Spinach and Feta
- **Lunch:** Quinoa and Roasted Vegetable Bowl
- **Dinner:** Vegetable and Chickpea Stew
- **Snack:** Roasted Almonds with Cacao Nibs
- **Dessert:** Baked Cinnamon Apples with Walnuts
- **Beverage:** Green Tea with Mint

Day 30:

- **Breakfast:** Avocado Toast with a Side of Berries
- **Lunch:** Mediterranean Hummus and Veggie Wrap
- **Dinner:** Grilled Salmon with Steamed Broccoli
- **Snack:** Rice Cakes with Avocado and Tomato
- **Dessert:** Lemon Poppy Seed Muffins

- **Beverage:** Cucumber and Lemon Infused Water

This plan provides variety while adhering to the guidelines of a low-histamine diet. The meals are nutrient-dense, focusing on whole foods like vegetables, lean proteins, and healthy fats. Enjoy!

Shopping Tip: Stick to the outer aisles of the grocery store, where fresh produce and meats are typically located, and avoid processed or pre-packaged foods that may contain hidden histamine triggers.

By planning ahead and following this guide, you can ensure that your low-histamine diet remains balanced and varied while managing your condition effectively.

Living with a low-histamine diet is a journey that requires ongoing preparation, self-care, and support. With the right approach, you can thrive while managing histamine intolerance.

Conclusion

As we reach the conclusion of Beginner's Guide to Low-Histamine Diet, I hope you have gained valuable insights into preparing nourishing and wholesome meals tailored to your specific dietary needs. While transitioning to a low-histamine diet may feel overwhelming at first, know that you are not alone. This guide is here to support you, providing the knowledge and tools you need to take control of your health and well-being.

Above all, always remember that you are cherished, and your choice to embark on this journey reflects your dedication to improving your health and vitality. By making thoughtful food choices, you are taking a meaningful step toward enhancing your taste buds and overall wellness.

I am grateful for your commitment and the trust you have placed in this meal guide. May the wisdom and recipes within these pages serve as a valuable resource to help you create a balanced, vibrant, and healthy life.

Wishing you the best on your path to renewed health, happiness, and vitality!